The Ultimate Guide to Easy Calisthenics for Beginners

Joshua H. Thompson

<u>***Funny helpful tips:***</u>

Life's adventure beckons; step forward with courage, curiosity, and joy.

Stay ethical in all business dealings; integrity builds trust and reputation.

*The Ultimate Guide to Easy Calisthenics for Beginners :
Unlock the Secrets of Effortless Calisthenics: A Comprehensive
Beginner's Handbook for Achieving Fitness Success*

<u>**Life advices:**</u>

Prioritize books that teach soft skills; understanding human behavior and emotions is invaluable in all life areas.

Protect your intellectual property; it's a valuable asset.

Introduction

This is a comprehensive guide designed to introduce individuals to the world of calisthenics and help them embark on their fitness journey. Calisthenics is a form of exercise that utilizes bodyweight movements and requires minimal equipment, making it accessible to people of all fitness levels.

The guide begins by explaining the concept of calisthenics and its benefits. It emphasizes the importance of diet and nutrition in supporting one's fitness goals and overall health. Readers are encouraged to understand their body and its capabilities before diving into the exercises.

The guide places great importance on proper warm-up and preparation to prevent injuries and improve performance during calisthenics workouts. Flexibility and stretching exercises are also included to help readers enhance their range of motion and maintain flexibility, which is vital in calisthenics movements.

The heart of the guide lies in the exercises section, where readers will find a range of upper body, lower body, and cardio conditioning exercises. The upper body exercises focus on building strength in the arms, chest, shoulders, and back. The lower body exercises target the legs and core, essential for overall stability and balance. The cardio and conditioning exercises help improve cardiovascular health and endurance.

Each exercise is described with clear instructions and illustrations to ensure proper form and execution. The guide emphasizes the importance of starting with basic variations for beginners and progressing to more challenging exercises as one's strength and skill improve.

Throughout the guide, safety tips and precautions are provided to ensure that individuals engage in calisthenics in a safe and effective manner. The importance of listening to one's body and avoiding overexertion is emphasized to prevent injuries and achieve long-term fitness goals.

With this book, readers are equipped with the knowledge and tools needed to begin their calisthenics journey. The guide provides a structured approach to building strength, flexibility, and cardiovascular fitness through bodyweight exercises. Whether readers are new to fitness or seeking an alternative workout routine, this guide offers a solid foundation to get started and progress in calisthenics.

Contents

1. WHAT IS CALISTHENICS?

If you're reading this book then the chances are you've already looked into calisthenics, probably read a few articles online and watched some videos of seemingly superhuman feats of strength by famous practitioners on YouTube.

These guys have it all; traps that reach up to their ears, sculpted shoulders, bulging chests, forearms like Popeye, abs you could grate cheese on and legs that could propel them to the moon. And all without pumping iron? Well, pretty much.

HOw DOES IT WORK?

Calisthenics, by definition, is a form of exercise that consists of various gross motor movements using your own bodyweight for resistance, normally without equipment or apparatus, with the exception of basic items such as a pull-up bar or parallettes.

This is the art of training your body as nature intended; not by isolating muscle groups and using complex man-made machinery that you would never find out in the real world, but by using the tools you are already equipped with. With calisthenics, your body is your gym, and the world is your playground.

WHAT DOES IT DO?

Calisthenics is the art of strengthening your entire body as a unit, eliminating each weak link in the chain until every fiber of your being is working in total harmony to produce extraordinary levels of strength.

Training like this achieves results you can use in the real world. Think about it, how often do you need to bicep curl something, or flap cables around over your head in everyday life? These are all man-made inventions designed to make single muscle groups strong IN THE GYM, but as soon as we step outside it becomes somewhat irrelevant.

To perform at maximum capacity in everyday life, or to acquire formidable strength and fitness for your sport, you need to be strong everywhere, not just in certain places.

Calisthenics strengthens every muscle group and every link between those muscle groups. It is the ultimate form of exercise for creating true strength that you can use every day, whether it be for regular tasks, your favorite sport or just showing off!

WHO IS IT FOR?

The simple answer to this question is that calisthenics is for everyone. Practicing bodyweight training can help anyone achieve a stronger, fitter, more flexible body.

Whether you are a lean athlete wanting to pile on more muscle mass, a 200-pound bodybuilder seeking to get shredded, a kick boxer requiring greater range of motion or simply starting up with exercise for the first time, calisthenics is the ultimate solution.

Don't just take our word for it. Professional sports teams and global militias often utilize calisthenics for its explosive effectiveness and practical application. You can use your bodyweight to train any place, any time, making it the benchmark fitness solution for high level operators across the world.

Don't get stuck performing the same old isolated exercises in the gym for years on end, choose calisthenics and take your gym with you wherever you go!

HOw CAN I GET STARTED?

One of the great advantages of calisthenics is that it's super simple to get started. You don't need a gym membership or any prior experience, and you can begin with simple exercises today.

With that in mind, here's a few key tips to make life easier for those just getting started:

1. Use a credible guide: This is your starting point! Don't dive straight in and use guesswork to correct course, as this often ends in disappointment or, worse, injury. Whether you choose to follow this guide or something else, the most important thing is that you stick to it like glue, and let the experts guide you to success.

2. Establish a program: Training without a program is like driving around a strange place without a map. In order to stay on track and keep up to date with your progress, you need a schedule. You can get one at the back of this book, or work with a trainer to create your own.

3. Get a training partner: Tests prove that accountability is a hugely effective catalyst for increasing performance. For us, this means getting a committed training partner and supporting each other on the journey.

Above all, starting up is as simple as putting on your sweats and getting out there. So, step up and step out, companion, it all begins here!

"There are no limits. There are only plateaus, and you must not stay there, you must go beyond them."

Bruce Lee

2. DIET AND NUTRITION

We can practically hear some of you screaming, 'I know what to eat, just get to the good stuff already!'

Well, we're going to shut you down like a rat-infested restaurant right now because diet and nutrition are the foundation of a great body and it would be a dereliction of duty to neglect this area.

If you want to maximize your results then don't skip this part.

HYDRATE

Water is life. We need it to transport vital nutrients around the body and to keep our muscles and minds functioning at full capacity.

Most people simply do not drink enough water day-to-day, which means both their performance *and* their recovery is greatly impaired.

According to The European Food Safety Authority, men should be drinking about 2 liters of water per day while women should get about 1.6 liters. This is, of course, a general guideline but if you are not hitting these figures you may be affected by dehydration. We recommend speaking to a physician or nutritionist to discuss your requirements.

If you are taking a supplement such as creatine, which affects the way that your body processes water, then you will need to drink more. Check out the label on all of your supplements and always ensure you take on board enough fluids.

While we're on the topic, steer clear of alcohol and fizzy drinks if you want to get ripped. They're packed full of carbs and sugar, and won't do you any favors whatsoever.

EAT RIGHT

Your particular goals will determine your diet, but there are some general guidelines to follow here if you want to get in the best shape possible.

Eat clean: We're not asking you to become a hippy or go plucking fruits from trees, but it really pays to cut out processed food and other junk.

Check the labels and pick up fresh foods which contain a single ingredient – i.e. whatever it is actually supposed to be – rather than something packed full of preservatives and lord knows what else.

Mix it up: You've heard it said over and over and now you're going to hear it once again; a balanced and varied diet is the key to good health. This means a mixture of proteins, carbohydrates and fats. Check out the following examples for some inspiration:

Proteins: Organic meat, poultry, fish, eggs and dairy are primary sources of protein.

Carbohydrates: Fruits and vegetables are a great source of healthy carbohydrates, as are sweet potatoes, wholegrain pastas, brown rice and similar grains.

Fats: Forget the myth of fat being bad for you. The type found in good quality meats, nuts, seeds, fish and olive oil is an essential part of your daily diet.

EAT FOR YOUR GOAL

When you strip diet and fitness down to their core elements it becomes very simple. If you want to gain weight and muscle mass, you simply have to eat more calories than you burn off.

If you want to maintain your weight and refine your body then you should be aiming to eat around the same amount of calories as you burn off. If you want to cut down then you should be burning off more calories than you are eating.

There are plenty of resources out there to assist you with your particular objective, but we would advise against obsessive calorie counting. Food should be something to look forward to and you will soon start to resent it if preparation becomes a chore. By all means use tools and technology to ensure you are on the right track, but don't beat yourself up over fractions of a gram.

With that said, you should be aware of your macros and make a conscious effort to meet them on a daily basis. If you're not sure what this means, it is essentially just the combination of fats, carbs and proteins which make up your diet. Everybody is different and only you can determine what is appropriate for your body and goals, but if you are unsure, it pays to contact a professional nutritionist for guidance.

Planning meals in advance and cooking in bulk is super useful here, as it cuts out the guesswork and reduces the risk of making poor decisions on impulse!

We could write a whole book on diet and nutrition, and perhaps we will, but this one is about calisthenics, so for now we must move on. Suffice it to say, though, that you should pay special attention to your diet and take the time to investigate it thoroughly in order to maximize your results.

"Looking good and feeling good go hand in hand. If you have a healthy lifestyle, your diet and nutrition are set, and you're working out, you're going to feel good."

Jason Statham

3. KNOW YOUR BODY

Think you know your body? Think again. It's one thing to isolate muscles with regular exercises such as the bench press or bicep curl but it is entirely another to employ whole groups at the same time to squeeze out that last gut-busting muscle-up or planche.

Putting yourself under such intense strain can be dangerous if you don't know what you are doing, so it is important to familiarize yourself with your body to ensure you are utilizing it correctly and not putting yourself at risk of harm.

We suggest keeping a body map handy. You'll find a basic one on the next page, but it's a good idea to take your learning further, otherwise you may have no idea what we mean when we discuss certain muscle groups.

There is no shortage of quality resources out there when it comes to biomechanics and the study of the human body, and the more you learn the more control you will have over your progress and results.

In addition to DIY textbook style studying, we always recommend hooking up with a qualified and reputable personal trainer or physician to assess your individual needs and goals, since we cannot be there to advise everyone in person.

Super important: If at any time you feel pain or discomfort during exercise, STOP. Try some slow, steady movements to test the area and stretch it out gently.

If pain persists or worsens, call it a day and seek advice on the issue. Refer back to the body map to hone in on the area and speak to a physician for further advice.

Only return to training when you can comfortably perform movements without feeling any pain or impingements. Do not be tempted to 'power through' an injury as this will only exacerbate the issue and delay your recovery time. It is much smarter to take a short break and get back on track quickly than to finish your session at the cost of weeks or even months out of action.

Remember, calisthenics may be completely different to anything you have performed before. You will likely awaken muscles you never even knew existed, and it is probably going to hurt like hell, so make sure you are suitably prepared.

To help brace your body for action we'll be covering warm-up and preparation next.

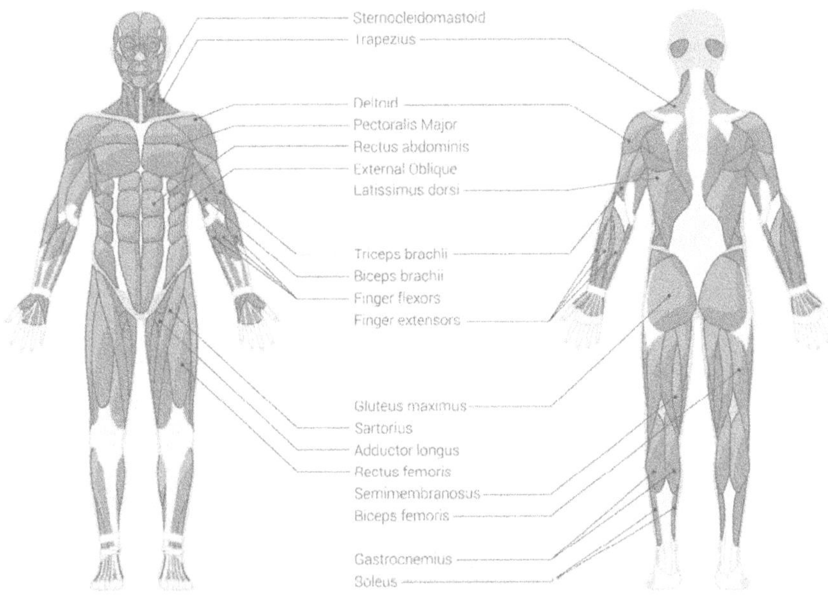

Above: A basic body map showing the major muscle groups. It is possible to drill down into much more detail, but we simply do not have the scope to cover everything in this guide. We highly recommend that you take your learning as far as time allows.

Remember, although we share the same basic physiology - with the exception of the obvious differences between the male and female anatomy - every individual is unique. Genetic factors beyond our control give us the blueprint with which we must work.

Instead of trying to 'fight' your genetics, we recommend working with them in order to sculpt your perfect body. If this sounds a bit heavy, don't worry, it simply means getting to know your strengths and weaknesses and working with those, instead of trying to force yourself down a path your body isn't prepared for.

That's not to say you can't build your dream physique, only that you should take a smart and informed approach. As always, we recommend speaking to a pro for more advice.

"Success is no accident. It is hard work, perseverance, learning, studying, sacrifice andmost of all, love of what you are doing or learning to do."

Pele

4. WARM-UP & PREPARATION

Whether you are a seasoned gym-goer or a complete newbie, calisthenics will shock your body to the core. You will awaken muscles you never even knew existed and aches and pains will spring up all over as you become stronger as a unit. For this reason it is essential to prepare properly if you want to achieve stunning results..

The benefits of warming up are threefold:

1. By getting the blood pumping and warming up your muscles you can hit the ground running and maximize performance during your workout.

2. You minimize the risk of getting injured during training, meaning you won't have to cut sessions short or drop out entirely due to niggles or tears.

3. Stretching helps you become more flexible over time, meaning you can increase your range of motion and subsequently push your body to new limits. As you scale up in this way you will gain unprecedented strength and capability.

Some people consider warming up to be a waste of time, but if you're not willing to put in an extra 5-10 minutes per session then we would have to question your commitment to calisthenics and fitness in the first place.

When you stop thinking of a warm-up as a chore and see the serious value it brings, it will revolutionize your workout and help you along the way to results you never thought were possible. But hey, don't just take our word for it.

Consider any of your favorite sports teams or stars. From professional football clubs to mixed martial artists, Olympic rowers to tennis players and everyone in-between, there is not a single person who steps out without some form of warm-up. If it's good enough for the greatest in the world, it's sure as hell good enough for us.

Remember: This book is focused on calisthenics, and while we can cover some essential mobility and flexibility exercises we simply don't have space for a complete solution. Use the following as a guideline and build your own warm-up routine over time. Add it to your routine and consider it sacred. Don't rush it, and don't skip it.

So, now that you understand the myriad of benefits warm-up and preparation brings to your workouts, let's get to work, shall we?

HANDS

In order to transfer maximum power from your hands to whatever piece of apparatus you are using you must ditch the gloves and go bare skin. This may seem somewhat counter-intuitive, because many gloves do offer additional exterior grip and most will make things more comfortable. Long-term, though, they will do more harm than good.

Consider pull-ups, for example. The extra layer between your hands and the bar means you are only as strong as your grip on the inside of the gloves. It doesn't matter how sticky the outsides are, because when that inner material starts sliding around, you'll drop like a sack of spuds.

So, the only way to transfer 100% of your energy to the bar is to make a direct and true connection. Your hands are going to take a battering and might feel sore at first but over time you will condition them to cope with these stresses and ultimately reap the rewards of a vice-like grip.

If you are using chalk or liquid chalk to help with your grip you might find your hands become very dry over time. Be sure to wash it off completely once you're finished and, if necessary, use a moisturizer.

You are unlikely to tear your hands apart when you are just getting started, but if for any reason you do cut them open don't act tough and carry on as this could put you out of action for weeks. It's best to rest for a day or two and let them heal before continuing.

Calluses are to be expected, but cuts and scars are not badges of honor to be worn with pride; they are a sign of bone-headed stupidity. Take care of your hands, and they will take care of you!

CARDIOVASCULAR

Once your hand preparation is taken care of, the first port of call in your pre-workout warm-up is to raise your heart rate and get the blood pumping.

Try 5-10 minutes of the following dynamic exercises to achieve this:

• Jogging, skipping, star jumps, cross-trainer, rowing

There are plenty of other ways to get your cardio fix, so mix it up a bit each day. Don't go overboard and leave yourself keeled over in exhaustion, but make sure it is intense enough to leave you a little out of breath. Your heart should be beating faster, and a light sweat is a good sign that you are ready to move on.

MOBILITY / MOTION

You've completed phase one of your warm-up, so the blood should now be pumping around your body, letting you know that you are ready to loosen up the areas you'll be hitting in your workout. We'll now run through some gentle mobility exercises designed to loosen up your limbs and increase your range of motion.

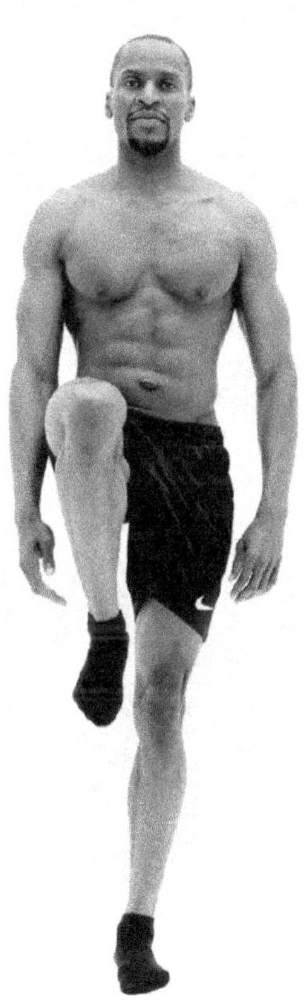

UPPER BODY

You will use every muscle fiber your upper body has to offer when training calisthenics so it is essential to get it ready for the task. Spend another 5-10 minutes going through the following, paying special attention to the areas of the body you plan to work out.

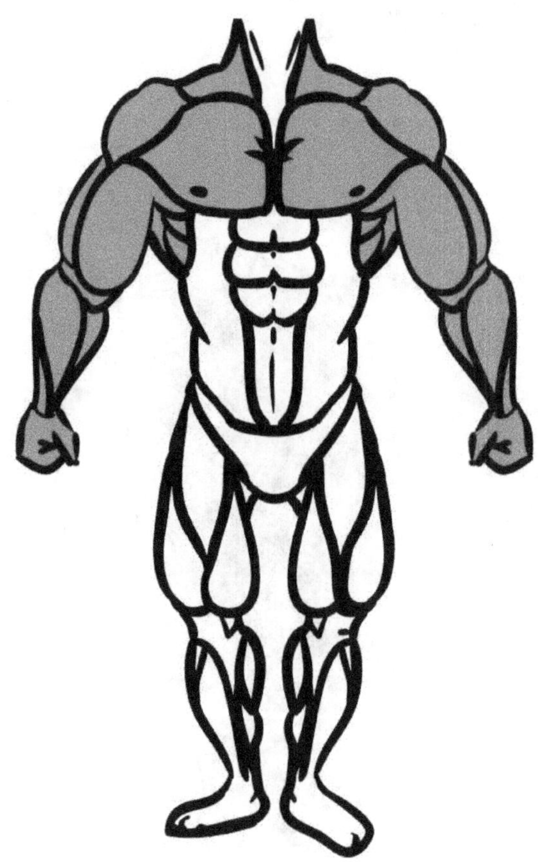

WRIST ROTATES

Your wrists are taxed in almost every calisthenics exercise, so try this simple warm-up to keep them strong and safe.

Perform: 10 seconds in each direction.

1. Extend your arms straight out in front of you.

2. Rotate your wrists clockwise for 10 seconds.

3. Switch directions and go again.

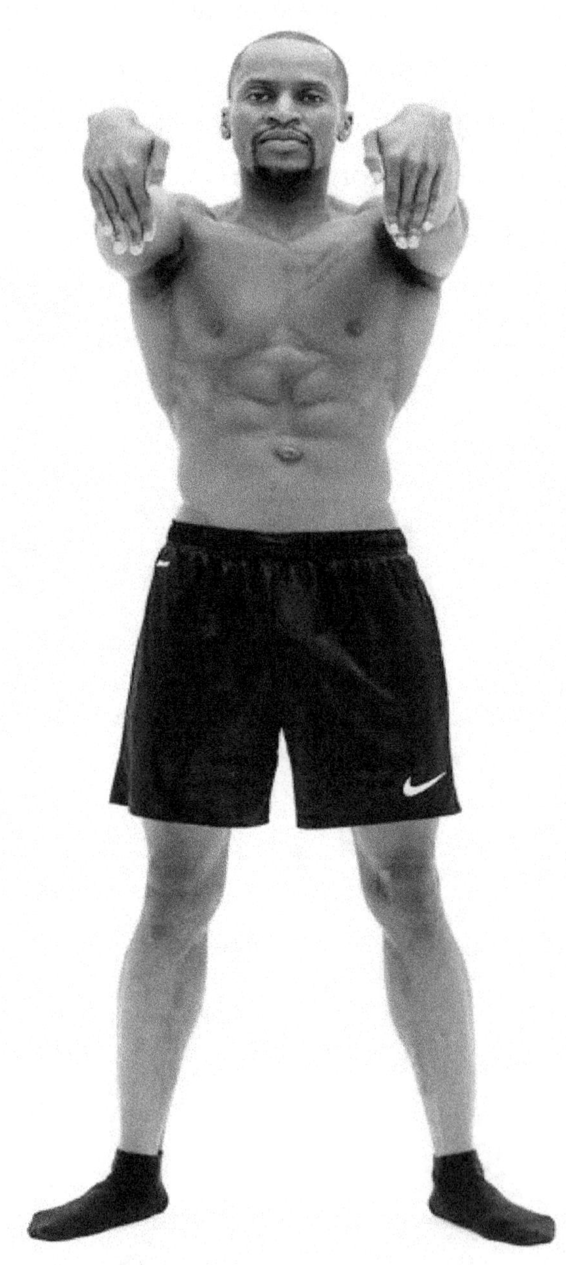

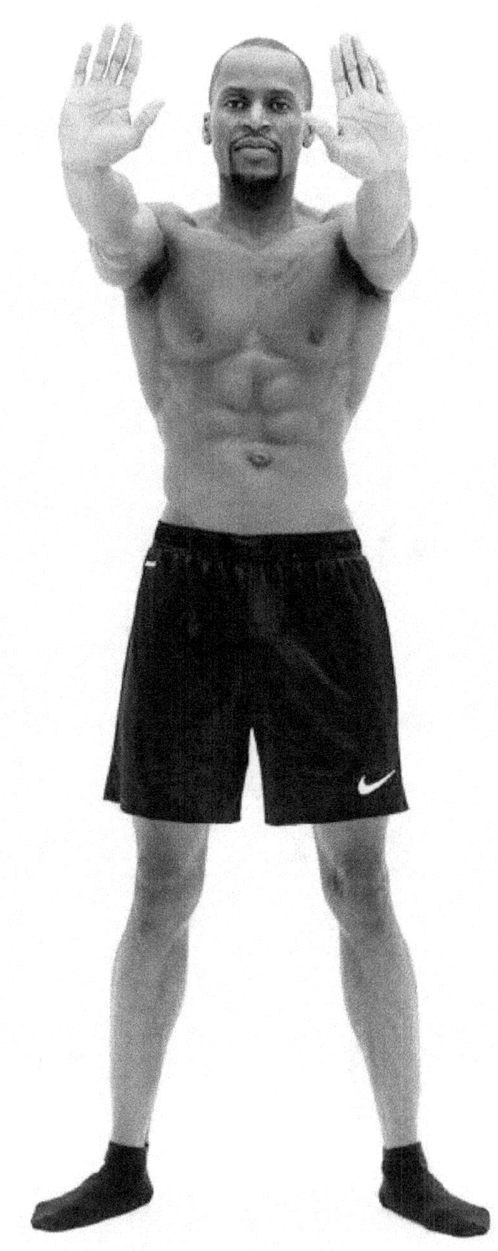

SHOULDER ROTATES

This is a simple but effective warm-up for the rotator cuff and shoulders.

Perform: 10 seconds in each direction.

1. Stand firm and extend both arms straight out to your sides.

2. Rotate arms forwards for 10 seconds.

3. Stop and do the same in reverse.

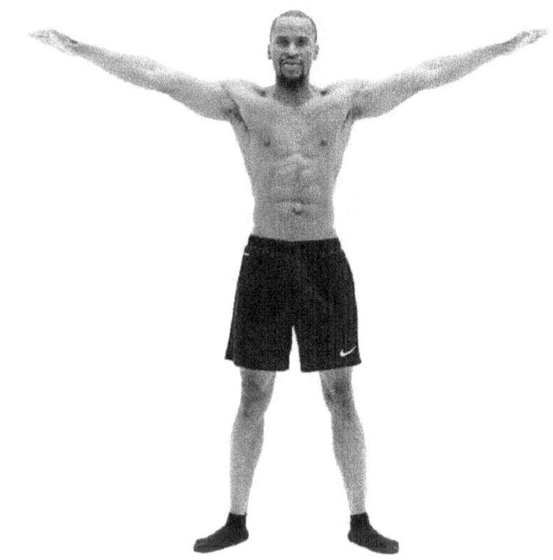

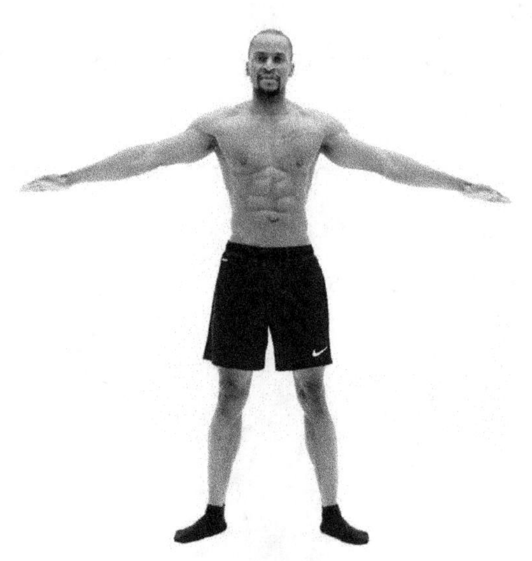

SHOULDER DISLOCATES

Don't panic, the clue isn't actually in the name this time! Your shoulders won't really pop out during this exercise, but they may still be a little uncomfortable at first. Since you will be opening up your shoulders, back, chest and arms here you will probably feel tightness in one or more areas.

Perform: 2 sets of 8 repetitions.

You will need: a long, lightweight bar.

1. Stand up straight, feet shoulder width apart, hands a little wider apart on the bar with an overhand grip (palms down).

2. Lift the bar up directly over your head and in one smooth motion bring it down to rest on your lower back, keeping your elbows locked at all times.

3. Reverse the movement, bringing the bar back to the front of your body to complete one rep.

You may struggle with this at first, so try sliding your hands wider apart along the bar until you find a position that allows you to perform the movement without bending your arms.

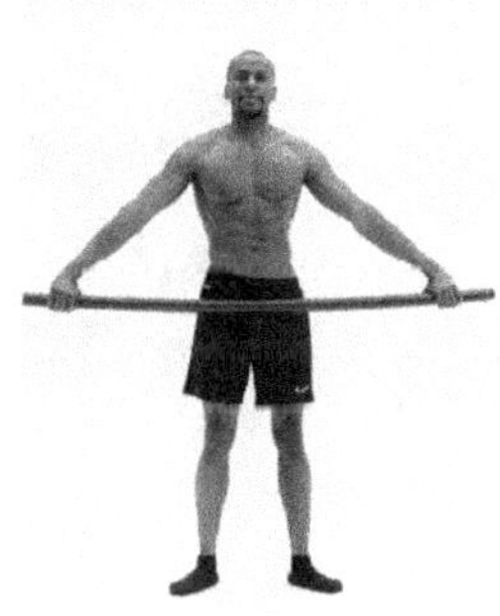

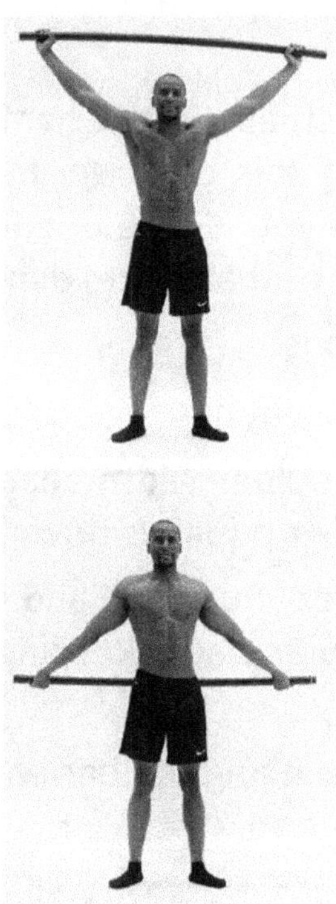

SCAPULA PUSH-UP

The scapula push-up is an excellent way to prepare your upper body for a beating. In particular, this will mobilize the muscles in your upper back and shoulders.

Perform: 8-10 repetitions.

1. Get into push-up position (see push-ups if unsure), placing your knees on the floor if you are just starting out.

2. Keeping your elbows locked and arms straight, let your chest sink towards the floor and squeeze your scapulae together at the same time.

3. With your elbows still locked, reverse this movement, lifting your chest back up and separating your scapula so that your back arches and your spine rises.

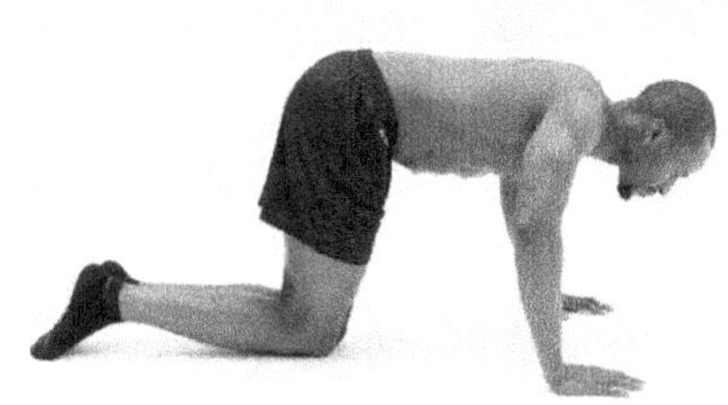

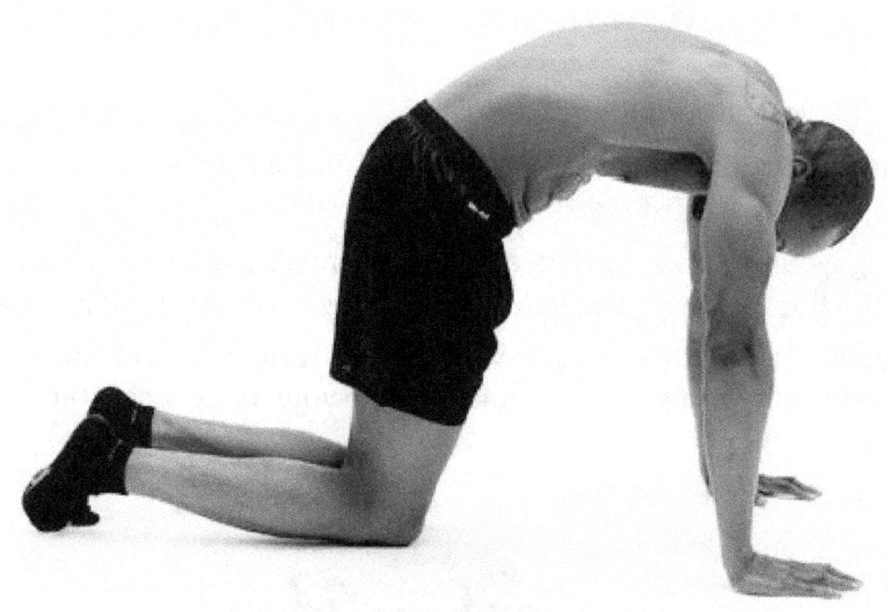

SCAPULA PULL-UP

The clue is in the name again; we'll be working your scapula and upper back here to great effect with an outstanding strengthening mobility exercise.

Perform: 8-10 repetitions.

You will need: a pull-up bar.

1. Grasp the bar overhand and allow yourself to hang with your arms and body totally straight, feet off the floor.

2. Relax, aiming to get your shoulders to touch your ears so your scapulae are elevated.

3. Keeping your arms and elbows locked in position; try to pull your scapulae downward.

4. Hold for 1-2 seconds and then lower back down to the starting position.

The movement involved in this exercise is so subtle that it is best demonstrated with good old-fashioned arrows! You may find this movement very difficult initially, but as with all things your mobility and control will improve over time so stick at it.

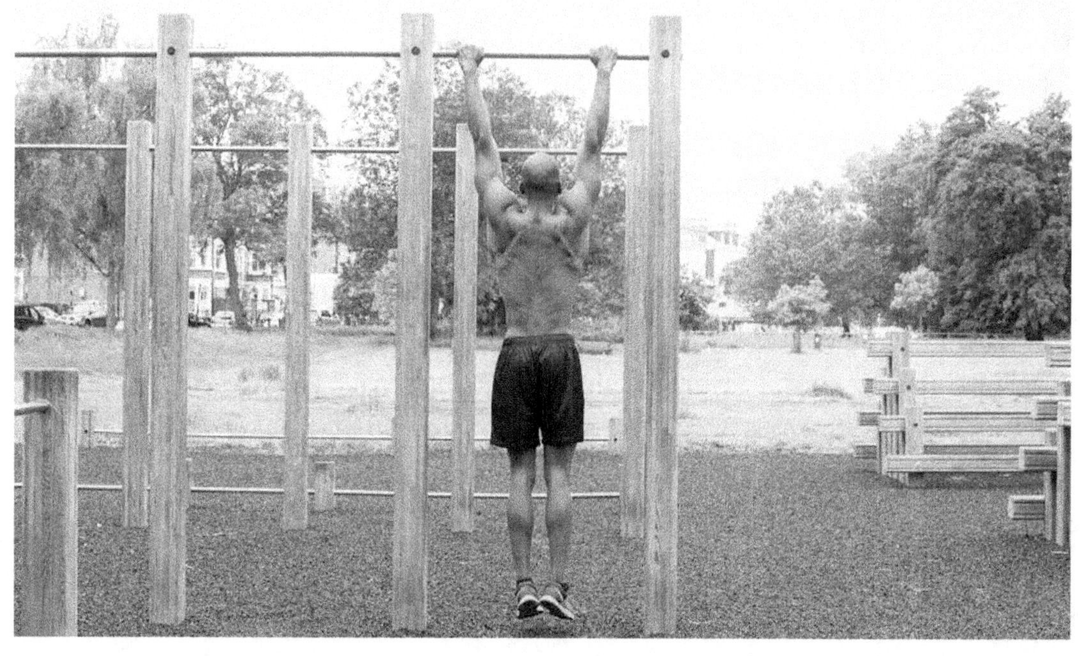

SCAPULA DIP

This motion will fire up your shoulders and give you greater range of movement for 'pushing' exercises such as, well, push-ups!

Perform: 8-10 repetitions.

You will need: parallel bars or dip station.

1. Grab the bars and lock your elbows, lifting your feet up and supporting your bodyweight in a neutral position.

2. Keeping your elbows locked and arms straight, sink your body down aiming to get your shoulders to meet your ears (or as close as you can).

3. With your arms still locked straight, push back upwards as high as possible, effectively trying to get your shoulders and ears as far apart as you are able.

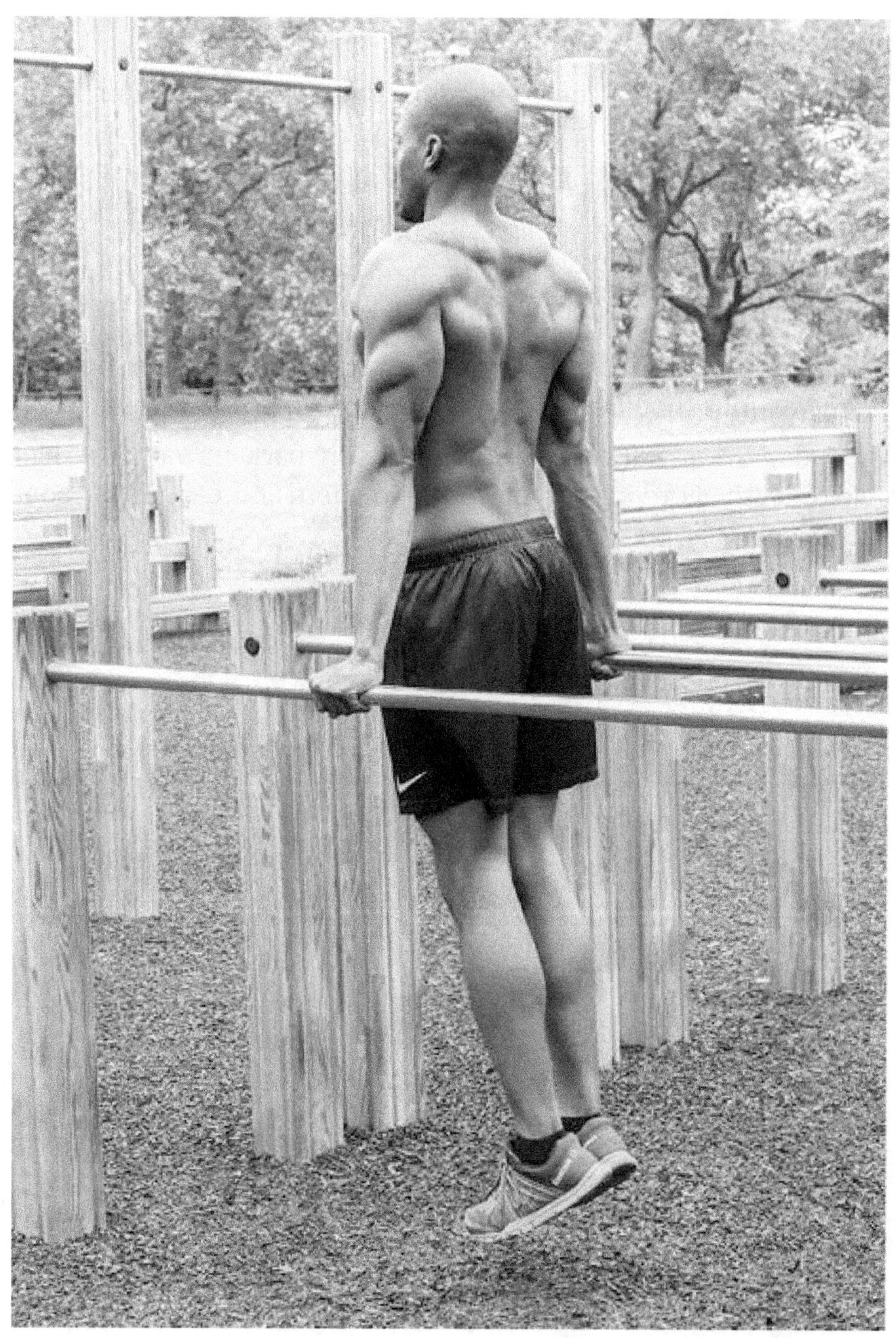

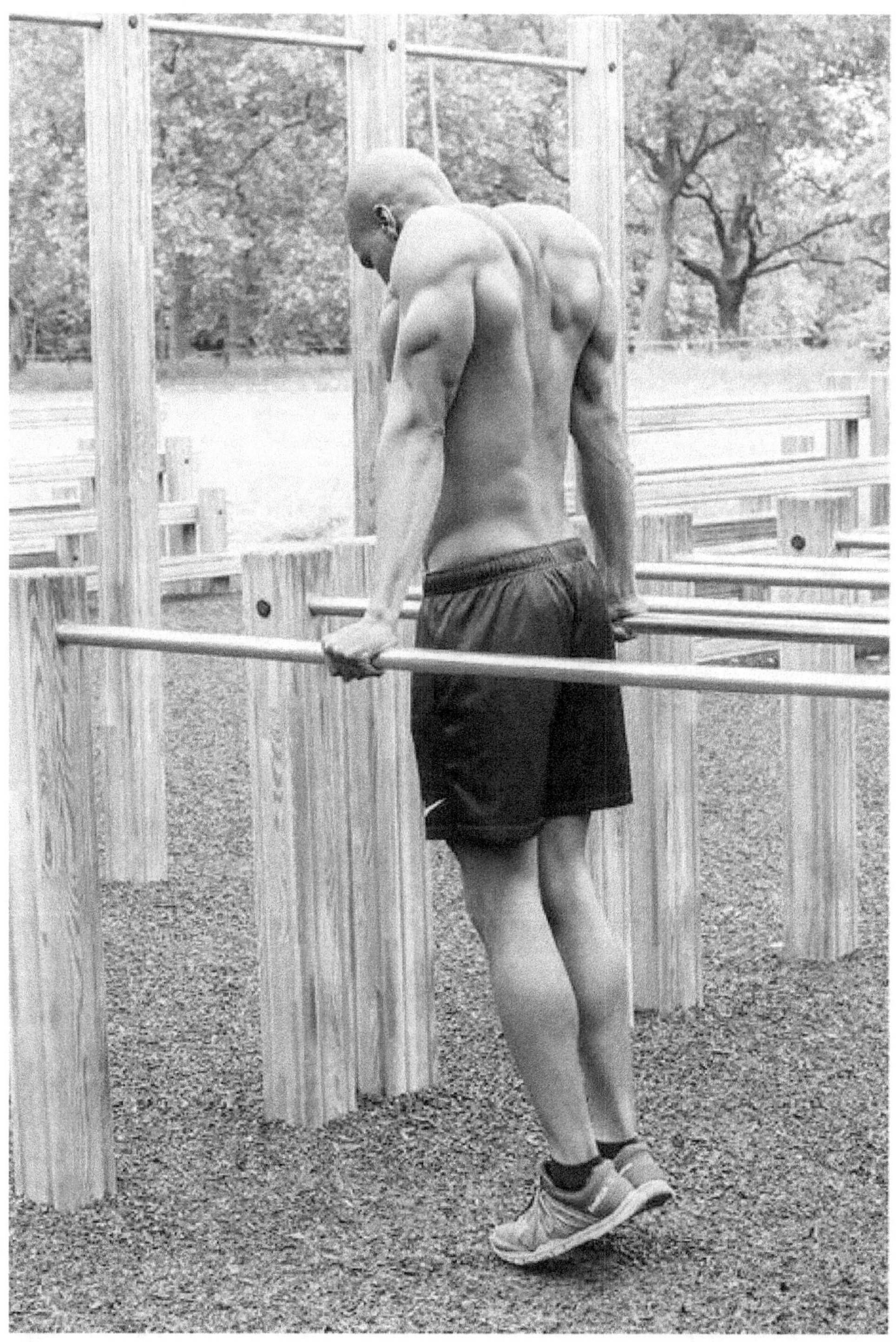

CORE

If you are taking your warm-up seriously then you should have broken a sweat by now. You will be glad to know that core mobility is nice and quick to address! Let's get to it.

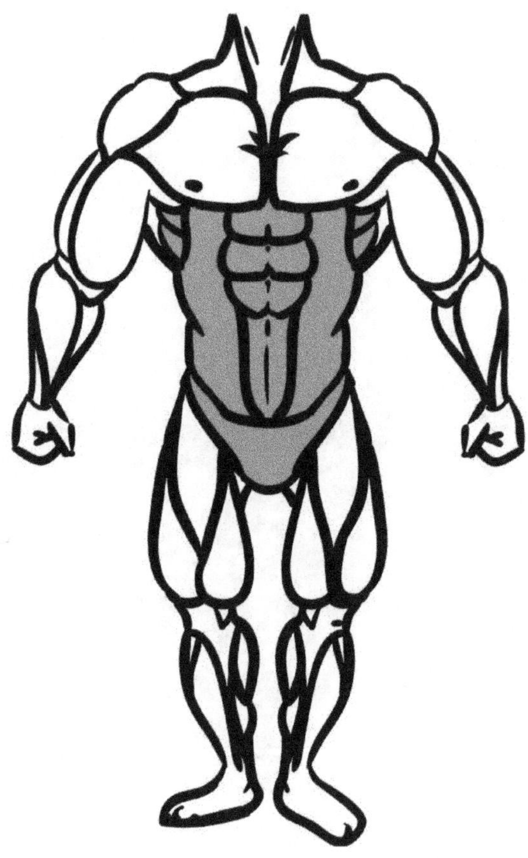

HIP ROTATES

Get your hula on to open up those hip flexors and increase your range of motion.

Perform: 2 sets of 8 repetitions in each direction.

1. Stand upright and place one hand on each hip.

2. Slowly rotate your hips clockwise in a 'hula' movement, aiming to keep your knees and back neutral, focusing the movement in your hips.

3. Repeat the movement counter-clockwise.

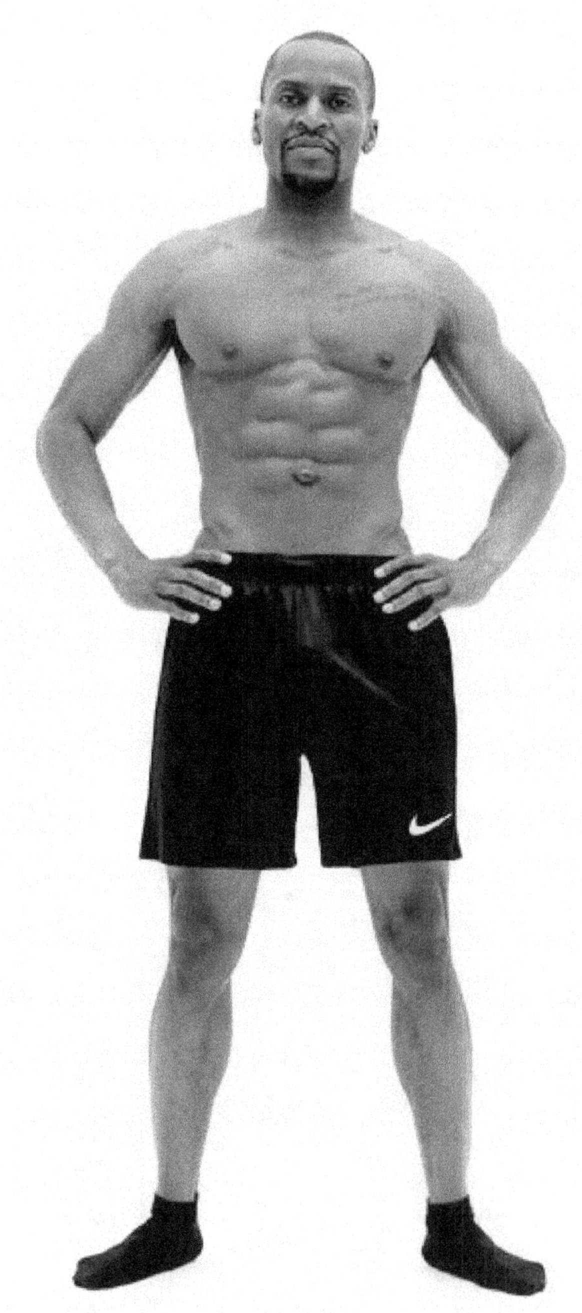

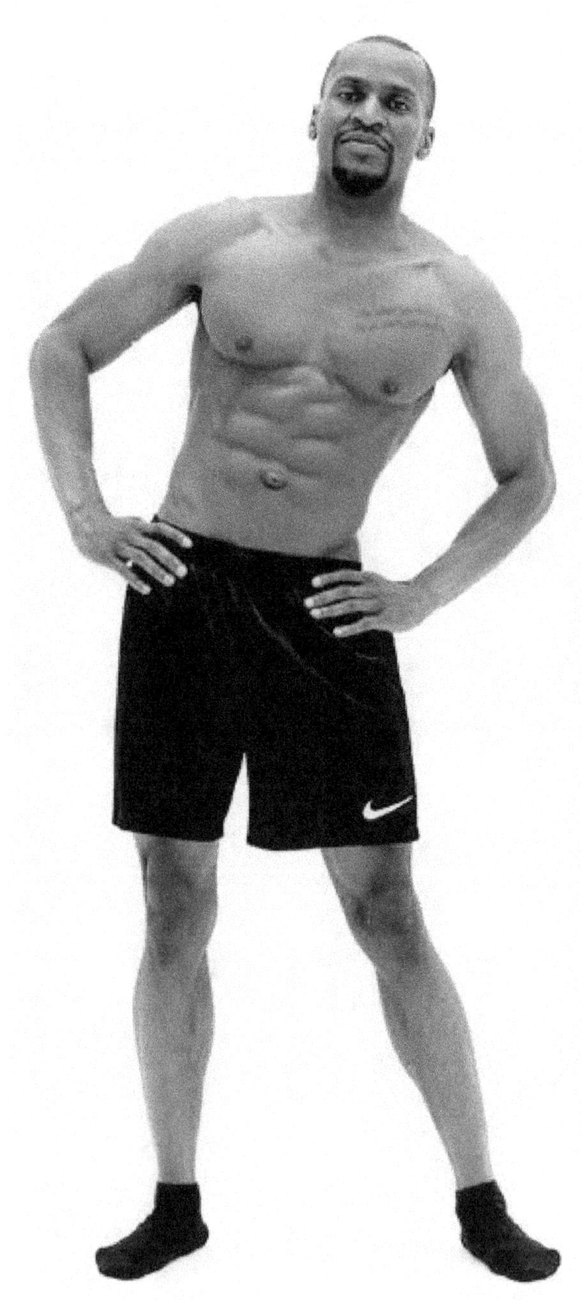

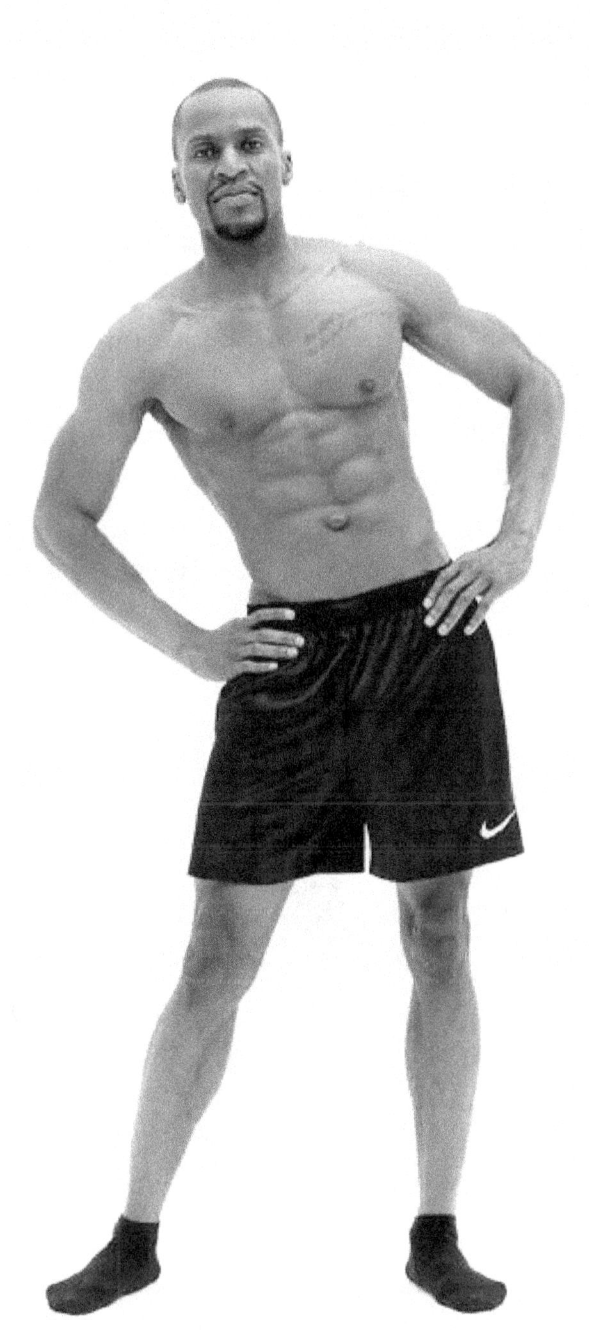

SIDE LEANS

Tight obliques and an inflexible lower spine can greatly inhibit your range of motion, so perform this movement to loosen up these areas.

Perform: 5 repetitions in each direction.

You will need: a long, lightweight bar.

1. Stand upright with your feet just wider than shoulder width apart, grasping the bar over your head.

2. Keeping your arms straight, feet rooted and shoulders in position, lean over to one side to stretch out the other.

3. When you have reached as low as possible, reverse the movement and repeat the exercise on the other side of your body.

Variation: You can perform this exercise without a bar if needs be, simply lean over to one side and grab your leg with the closest hand, bringing the other arm up overhead.

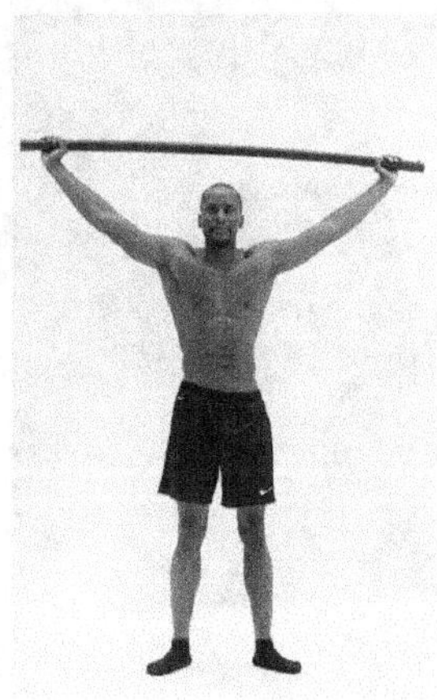

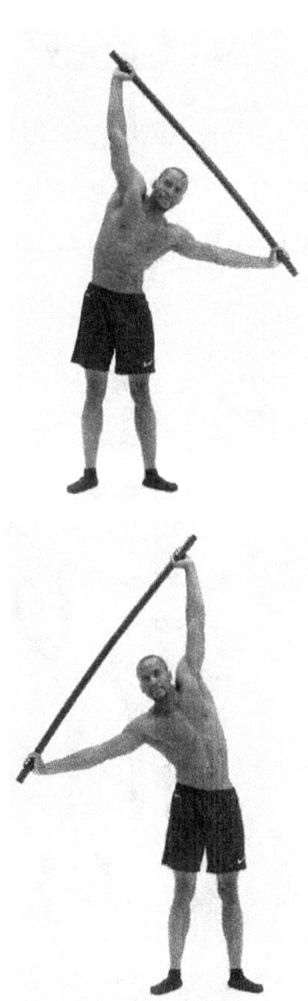

Even if you're not training lower body you will still be using it to get around so it's good practice to perform these exercises, too. Check out the following and incorporate them into your routine, or simply practice them on off days.

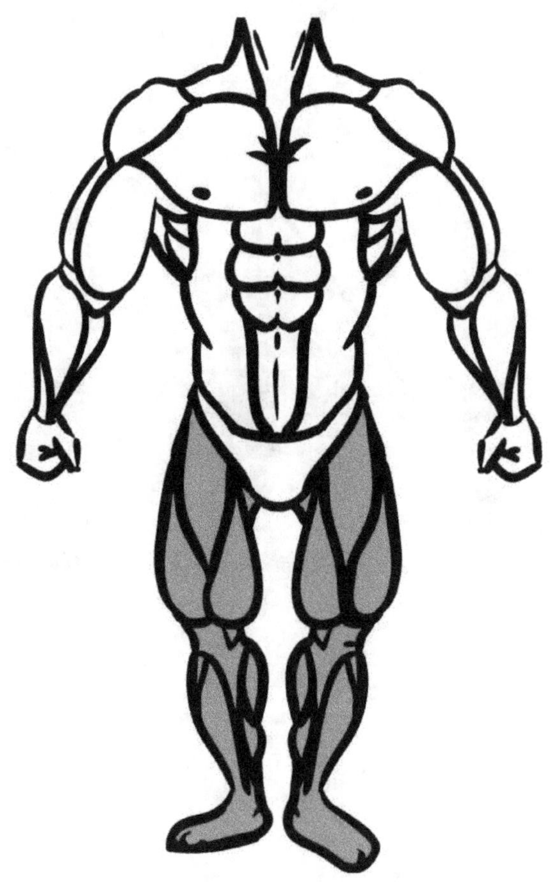

OPEN / CLOSE GATES

This is a staple mobility exercise for elite athletes across a whole range of sports, so it is well worth adding into your routine.

Perform: 8-10 repetitions on each leg.

1. Stand upright and raise one leg upwards, knee bent at 90 degrees.

2. Bring the leg out to the side to open up your hips and groin.

3. Perform the same movement in reverse, first bringing the leg up to the side, then around to the front and back down to the ground.

Variation: You can also perform this exercise on your hands and knees, lifting one knee off the ground, extending it backwards and then bringing it all the way back round the front, and vice versa.

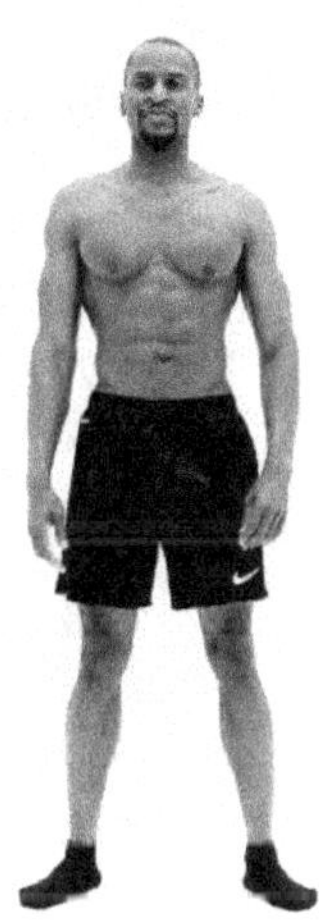

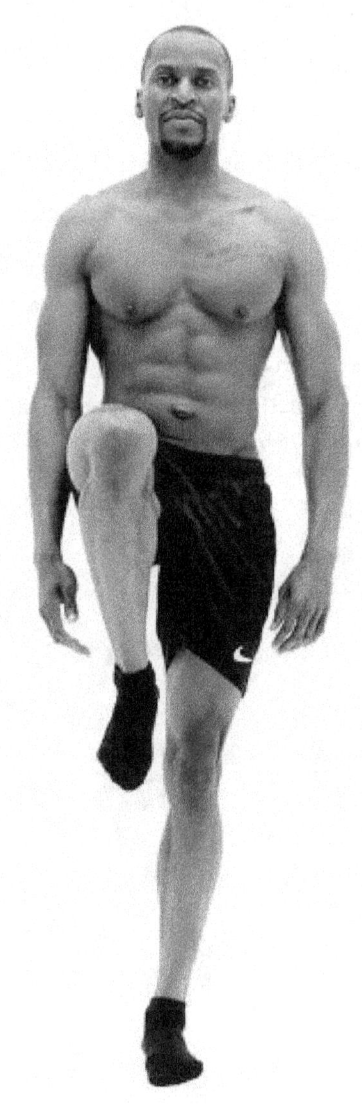

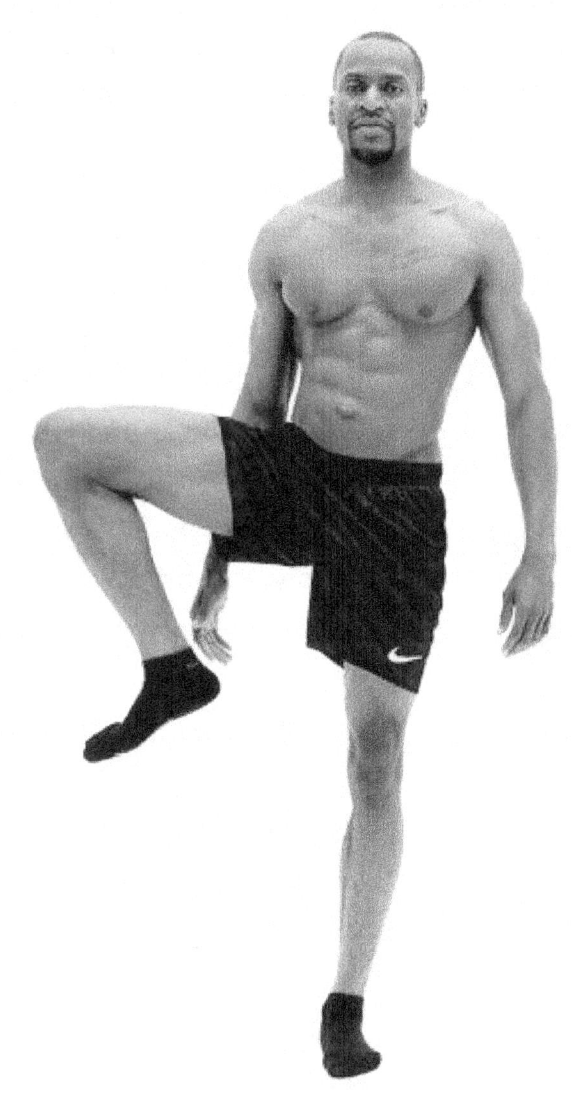

DEEP SQUAT

The squat is an exercise in itself, but we can make it – and almost every other lower body exercise – more effective by practicing the deep squat routinely. Because this one takes a little longer than the others you may prefer to do it on off days or after a heavy lower body session.

Perform: 3-5 minutes or more hold time.

1. Stand with your feet just beyond shoulder width apart, toes pointing out slightly at a comfortable, neutral angle.

2. Bend your knees and lower down into a squat position, ensuring you keep your lower back straight and push your hips back while doing so.

3. Once in position, clasp your hands together and rest your elbows just inside your knees, creating leverage to push your legs outward slightly.

4. Hold for 5 minutes, or as long as you can comfortably.

Variation: If you struggle to maintain your balance at first, place your legs either side of a sturdy pole or fixture and hold onto that to ensure you maintain the proper form.

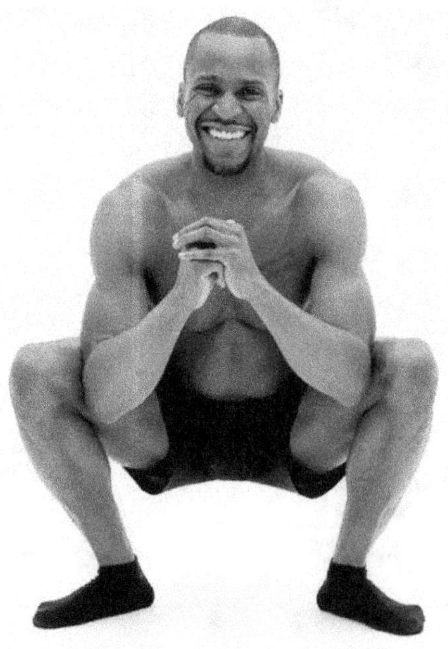

MOUNTAIN CLIMBERS

This is a fantastic, and dynamic, movement to warm up your body and get the blood flowing. Keep your reps unbroken and really lean into the movement to achieve the maximum benefit and increase your hip mobility.

Perform: 8 reps.

1. Assume the push-up position with your arms completely locked out, bringing your left leg forward and placing your foot beside your left hand.

2. Push both feet off the ground and quickly switch them. Now your right foot should be forward and your left out back. This counts as one rep.

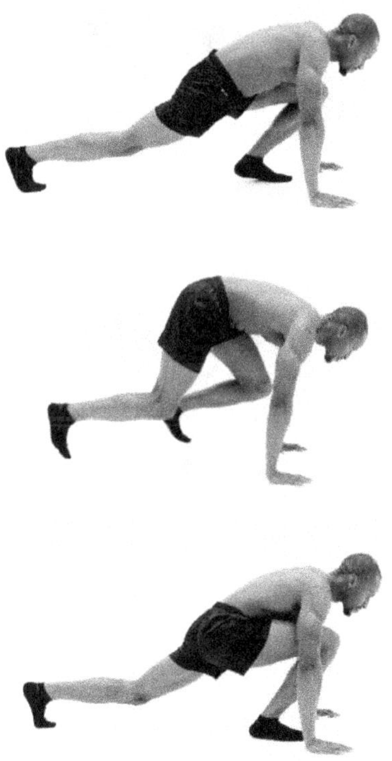

FROG HOPS

This is another excellent exercise to improve your hip mobility, and prepare your body for any exercise involving the lower body.

Perform: 8 reps.

1. Assume the push-up position with arms fully locked out.

2. Leave your hands in place, and jump forward with your feet, landing with them just outside your hands.

3. Reverse the movement and return to the start to complete one rep.

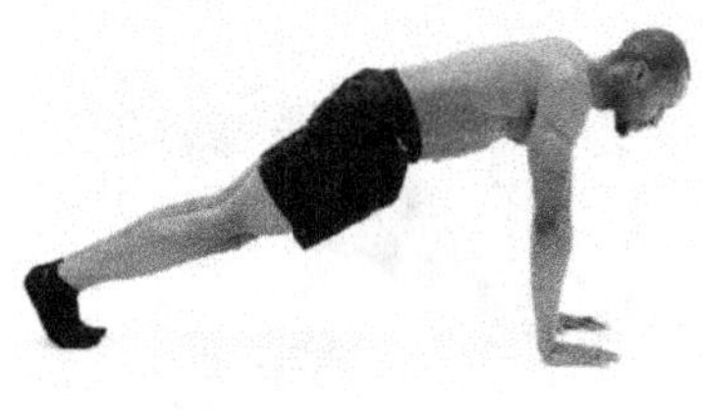

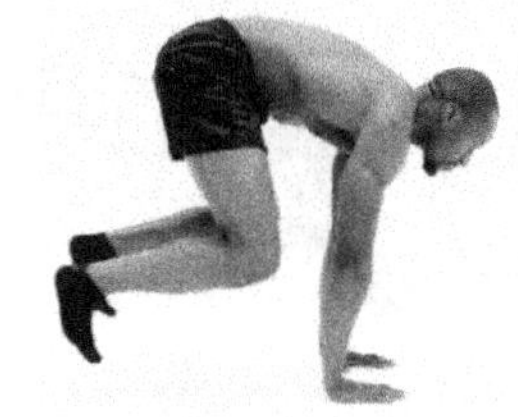

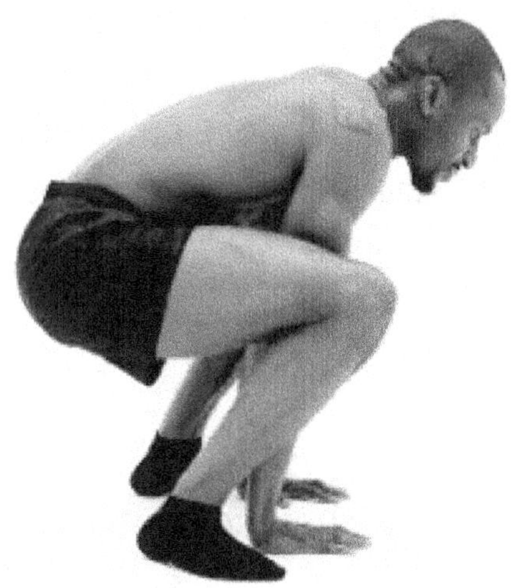

FLEXIBILITY & STRETCHING

Flexibility is a key component of a wide range of motion and, therefore, strength. Static stretching is the act of holding certain positions, generally for 15-30 seconds, in order to increase flexibility and minimize risk of injury.

You should be stretching after your workout or, if you are feeling tight in certain areas pre-workout, stretch them out then. Check out the following examples to target each area of your body. You can also do this on off days to accelerate your progress.

Remember: If you still feel tight in certain areas after stretching, throw in another set.

Tip: Relax during stretching. This might sound counter-productive but it is relaxing the muscles that allow them to stretch further. Try letting out a long, deep breath as you stretch a muscle and feel how much further it takes you!

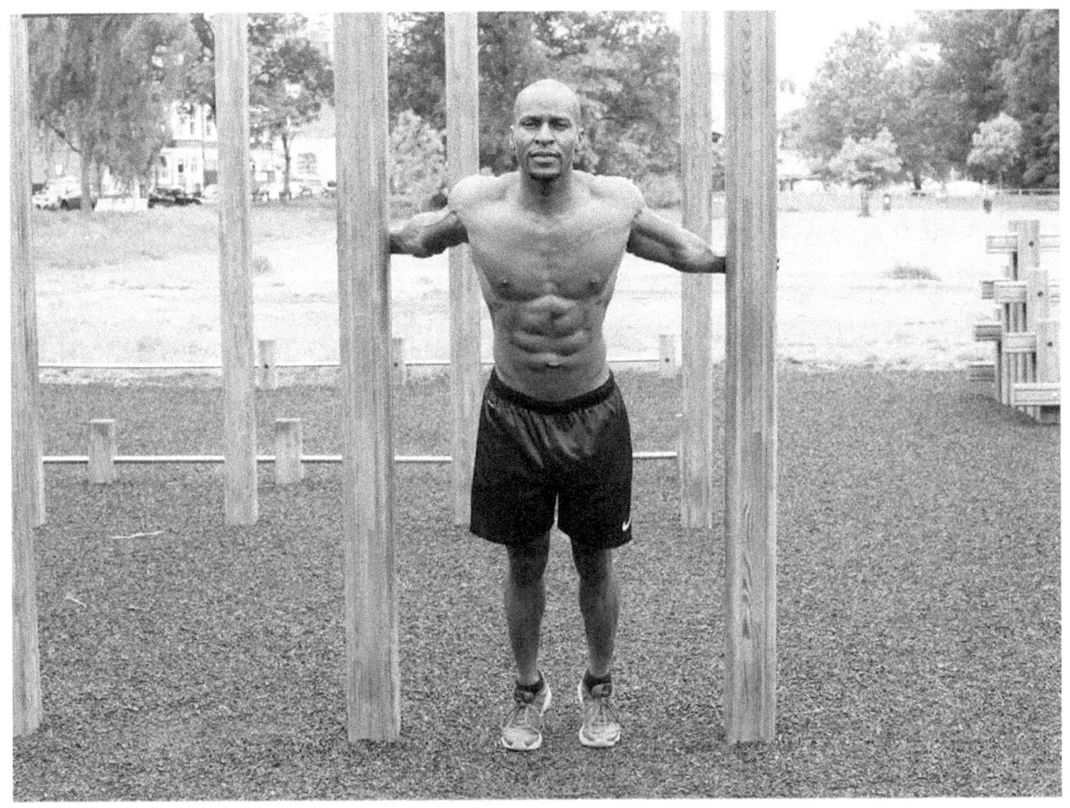

UPPER BODY

The upper body takes a beating during calisthenics training, so ensuring you are fully prepped is key. By improving your flexibility you will also get more out of your workouts, therefore enjoying greater results. We'll start from the top and work our way down.

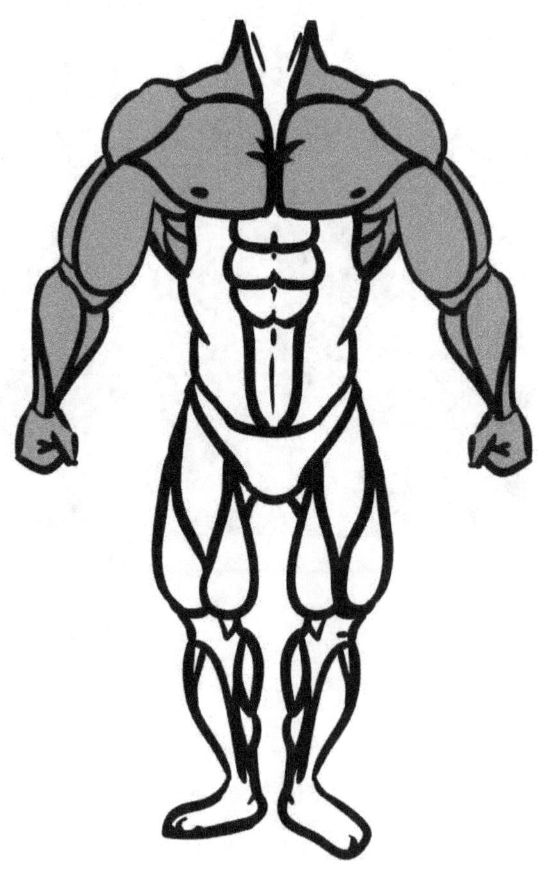

WRISTS & FOREARMS

Great as preparation for handstands as well as all-round strength, get to know both these variations to strengthen your wrists.

Perform: 30 second hold time.

1. Get on your knees and place your palms flat, fingers facing forward, just in front of your knees.

2. Lock your arms and slowly lean forwards as far as you can without raising your palms, and hold for the allotted time.

3. Return to start position and repeat the exercise, this time with your fingers facing towards you and leaning backwards instead of forwards.

Variation: If you find this too difficult then use a wall to perform a similar stretch.

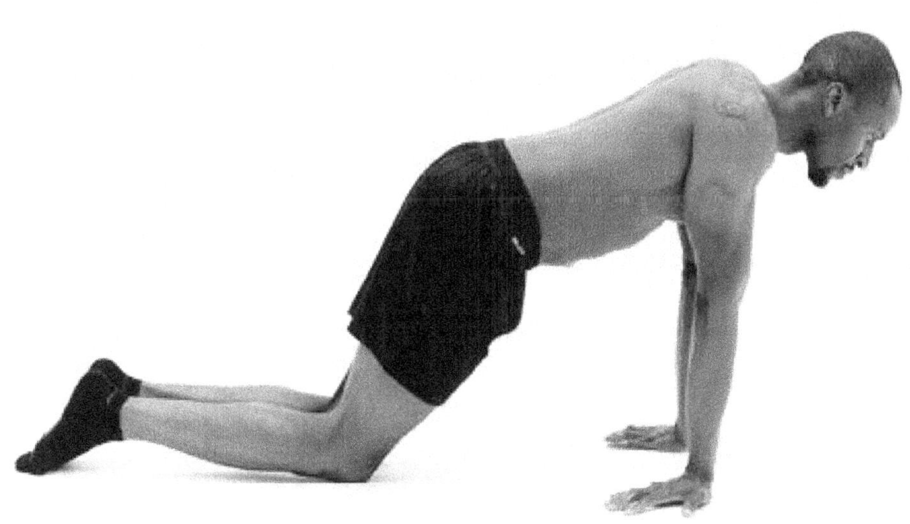

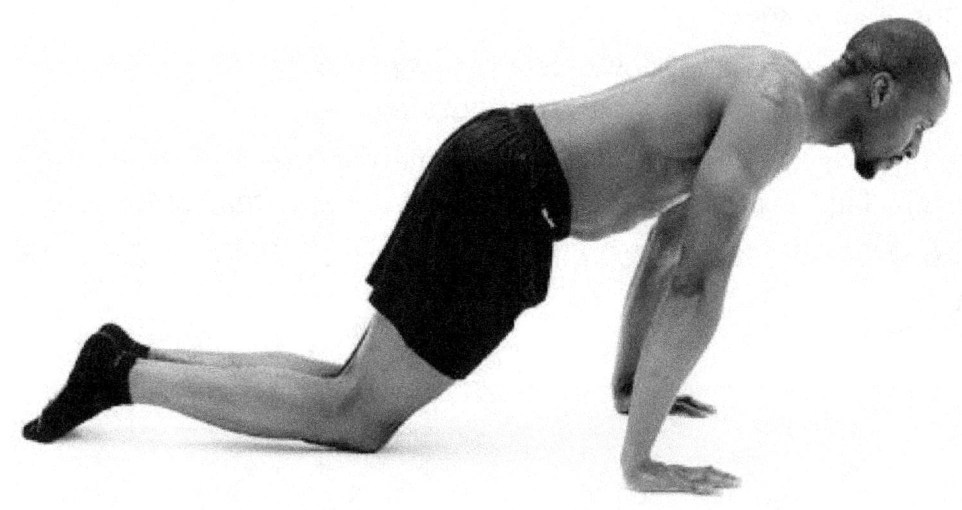

CHEST & SHOULDERS

This stretch is essential in opening up two of the largest muscle groups in your upper body. Find somewhere comfortable and relax into it.

Perform: 30 second hold time.

1. Get onto your hands and knees, then stretch your arms out in front of you.

2. With your hands and knees rooted to the spot, bring your chest down towards the ground, exhaling as you go.

3. When your chest and shoulders are as low as possible, hold this pose for the allotted time. Remember to relax.

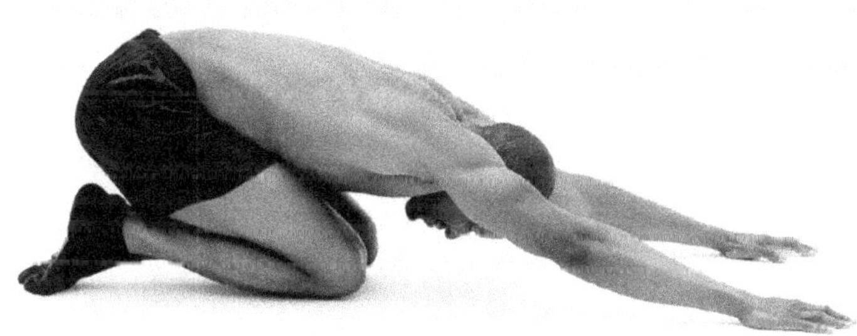

CHEST II

Your chest bears the brunt of almost every upper body exercise in calisthenics, so keep it properly conditioned with this simple stretch.

Perform: 30 second hold time.

You will need: upright parallel bars or doorframe.

1. Stand between the bars or doorframe and stretch your arms out to the sides, placing your palms flat on the surface.

2. Ensuring your arms stay straight, lean forward and stretch out your chest, holding for the allotted time.

Variations:

• If you don't have parallel bars use a single bar to stretch one side at a time. Instead of leaning forward, simply turn your body away from your affixed hand to stretch out one side of your chest then repeat on the other.

• You can also perform this exercise on a flat surface, rooting one hand against it and rotating away from that hand.

• Place a medicine ball or other platform on the floor and kneel beside it. Place one arm up on the platform, and then lower your body down to stretch out that side of your chest.

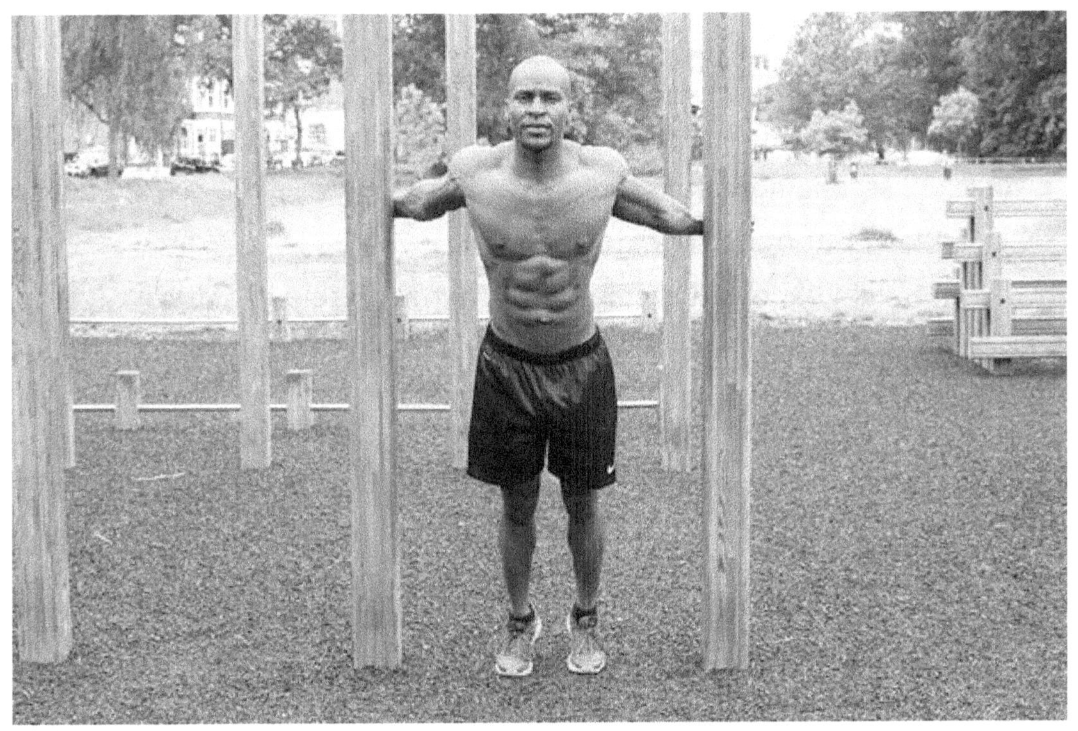

UPPER BACK

This is another area that will take a beating as you condition your body, so get into the habit of stretching it out.

Perform: 30 second hold time.

You will need: a study bar or fixture.

1. Grab a straight bar or other immovable fixture with one hand.

2. Keeping your arm locked, slowly lean back to stretch out your lattisumus dorsi (lat) on that side.

3. Bring your free arm around in front of your body to stretch further and hold for the allotted time. Repeat on the other side for an effective back stretch.

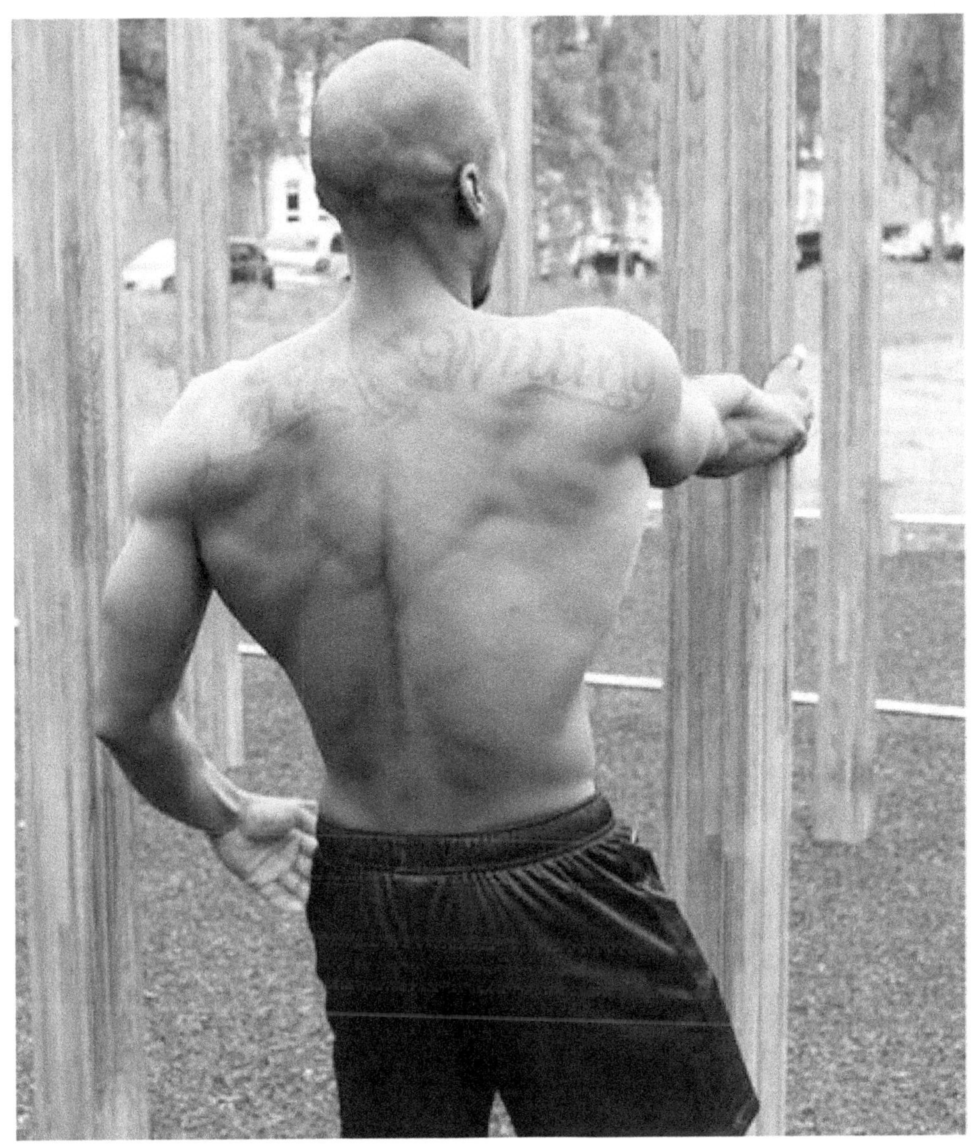

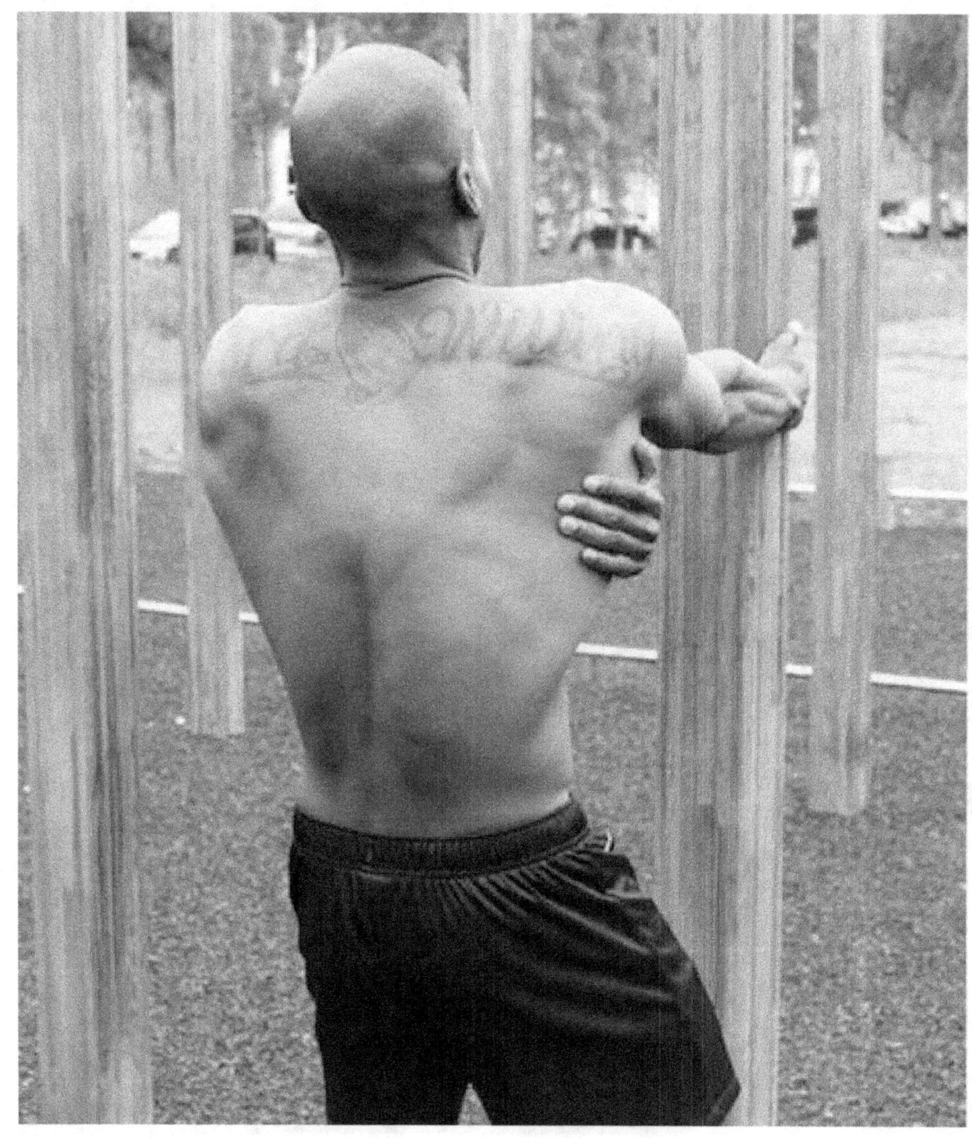

CORE

Everyone covets a chiseled core, and combining mobility and flexibility exercises with bodyweight training will help you achieve just that. You'll find this part quick and easy.

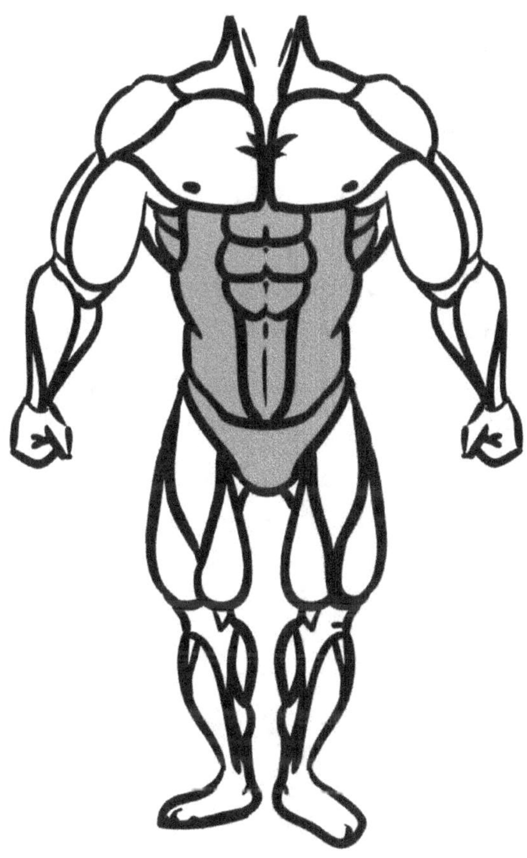

SIDE STRETCH

Prepare your lats, obliques, and lower back for movement with this standing side stretch, the same movement covered in mobility previously. As with all stretches, you don't want to be flexing, or straining against the movement. Instead, let your muscles relax and fall into the stretch for maximum benefit.

Perform: 15 second holds per side.

You will need: a long, lightweight bar.

1. Stand upright with your feet just wider than shoulder-width apart, grasping the bar over your head.

2. Keeping your arms straight, feet rooted and shoulders in position, lean over to one side to stretch out the other.

3. When you have reached as low as possible, reverse the movement and repeat the exercise on the other side of your body.

Variation: You can perform this exercise without a bar if needs be, simply lean over to one side and grab your leg with the closest hand, bringing the other arm up overhead.

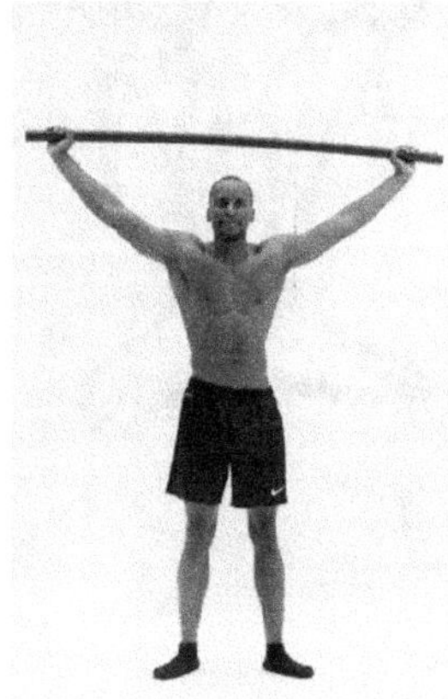

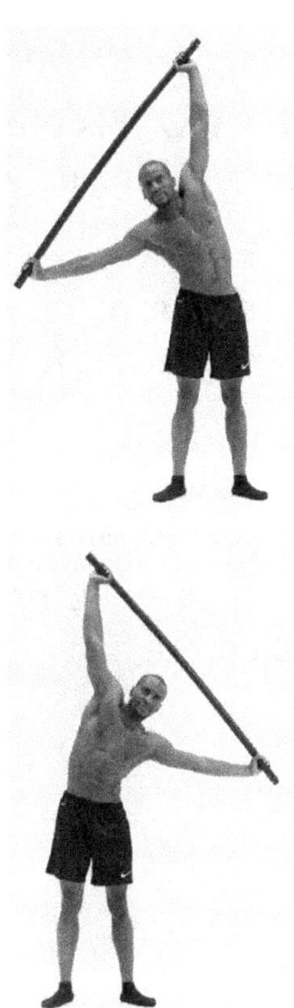

COBRA

If you've ever done yoga you'll know this one as the 'cobra' already. For everyone else, here it is, ideal for opening up your lower back and hips.

Perform: 15-30 second hold time.

1. Lie on your stomach and place your palms flat on the floor, similar to a standard push-up position, fingers facing forward, about shoulder-width apart.

2. With your hips rooted to the ground, raise your head and look upwards, allowing your spine to arch and hold for allotted time.

Variation: If you find this tough to hold, practice raising up onto your forearms and holding the stretch there first.

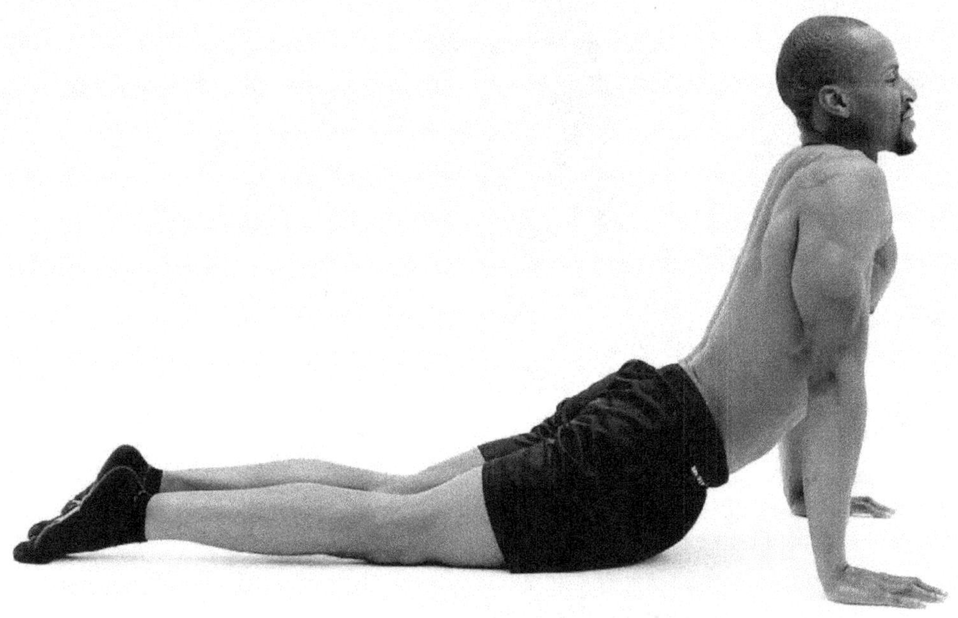

CAT

Another yoga stretch named 'cat', essentially designed to stretch the opposite way to cobra, opening up your back nicely.

Perform: 15-30 second hold time.

1. Get on your hands and knees, palms flat directly underneath your shoulders, fingers facing forward.

2. Drop your head and arch your back as if trying to look at your naval, and hold for the allotted amount of time.

Variation: To turn this into a mobility exercises, get into position and then transition to a downwardly arched back, raising your head up. Moving between the two in a fluid motion is a great way to warm up.

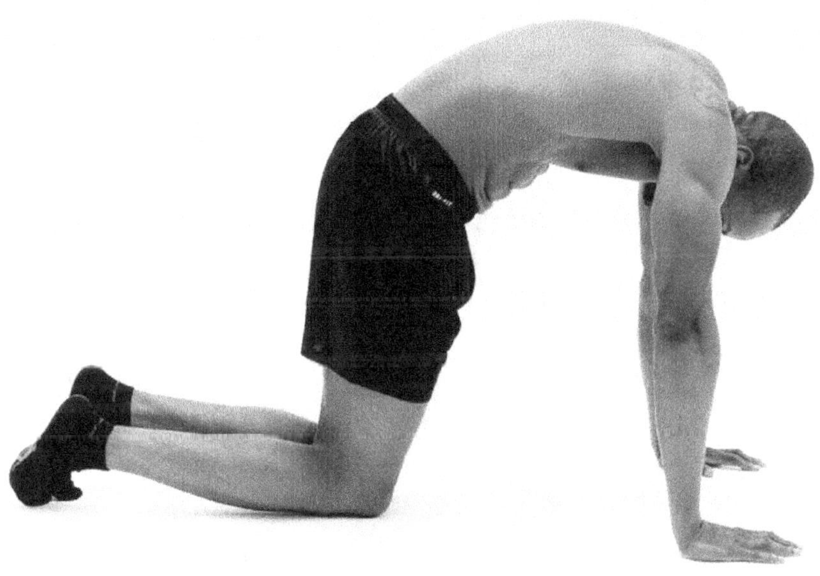

LOWER BODY

Last but by no means least is lower body flexibility. Not only will this help you achieve your dream body, it will also prove useful in everyday life, especially as the years go by. Don't let tight hamstrings, hip flexors or other problem areas hold you back. Let's go!

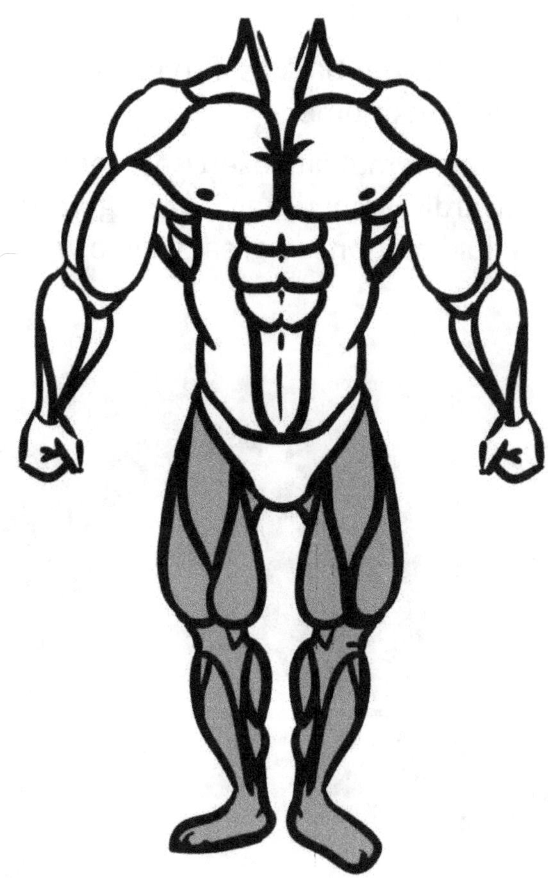

CALVES

Essential for strength and stability, you must ensure your calves are flexible enough to cope with the demands of calisthenics. And, of course, for showing off at barbeques!

Perform: 30 seconds hold time for each leg.

1. Get into push-up position.

2. Take one foot and rest the top of it on the heel of the other.

3. Slowly push the heel of the standing foot down as far as possible and hold for allotted time.

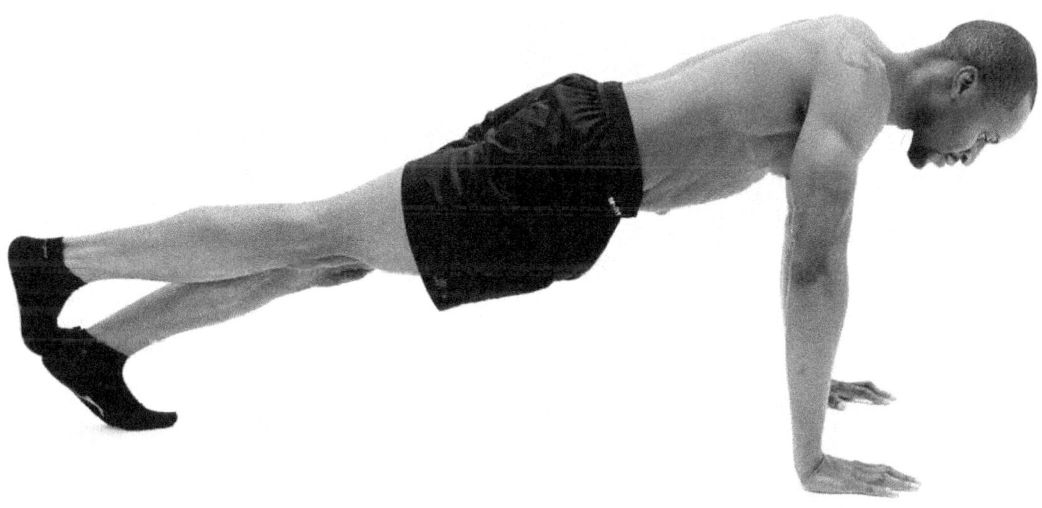

HAMSTRINGS

Most people have tight hamstrings, which can severely inhibit your range of lower body motion. Loosen them up like so:

Perform: 30 second hold time on each leg.

1. Sit down with both legs stretched out in front of you, toes pointing upwards.

2. Bring one foot towards you so the sole is against the inner thigh of the other leg.

3. Keeping your back straight, lean forwards towards the toes of your outstretched leg and hold for allotted time.

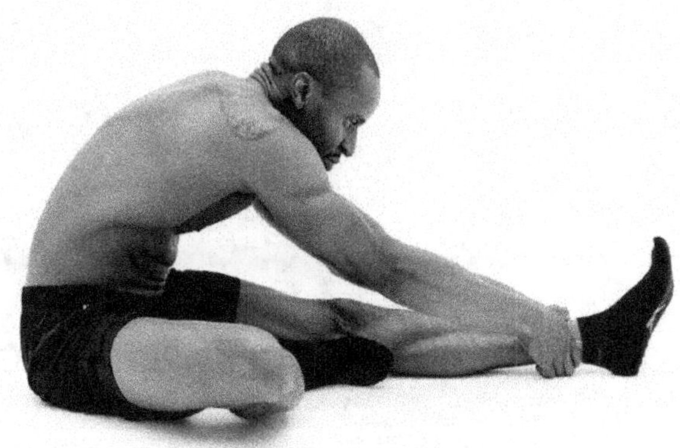

GROIN

Opening up your groin will also open up your hips. You are probably beginning to see how everything is linked together now, so you should never neglect one area in favor of another.

Perform: 30 second hold time.

1. Sit down and bring the soles of your feet together.

2. Keeping your back straight, pull your feet towards your body as close as possible.

3. Try to move your knees outwards to touch the floor. If you cannot do this with leg power alone, use your elbows or hands for a little assistance.

4. Hold for allotted time. You may find one side tighter than the other here, but don't worry, it will even out over time.

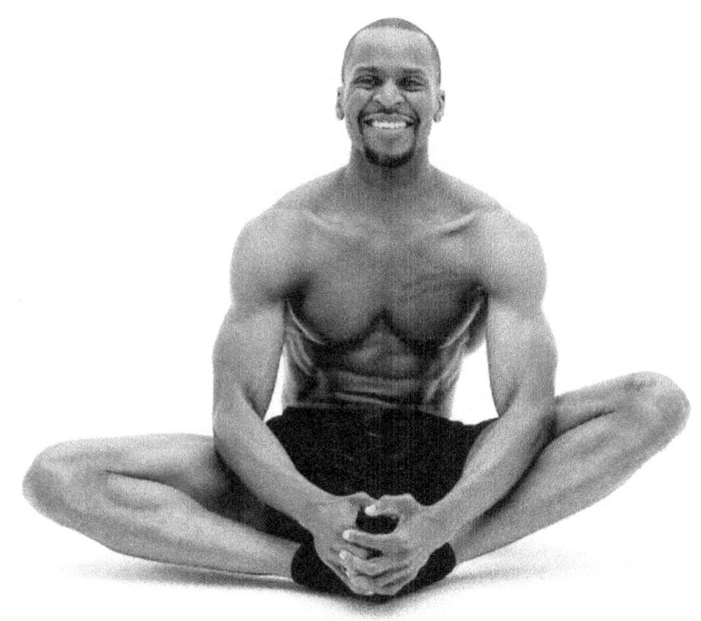

GLUTES

This is a hugely powerful part of your body, driving some of the most important motions required for lower body activities, which is why professional athletes and sports stars often have backsides like Beyoncé.

Perform: 30 second hold time on each side.

1. Lay on your back.

2. Bend the knee of one leg and bring it towards you, grasping the leg underneath your hamstring area with both hands.

3. Bring the other leg up and over so the ankle is resting just above the knee of the leg you are holding.

4. Pull the leg you are holding towards you to create a stretch in the opposite glute and hold for allotted time.

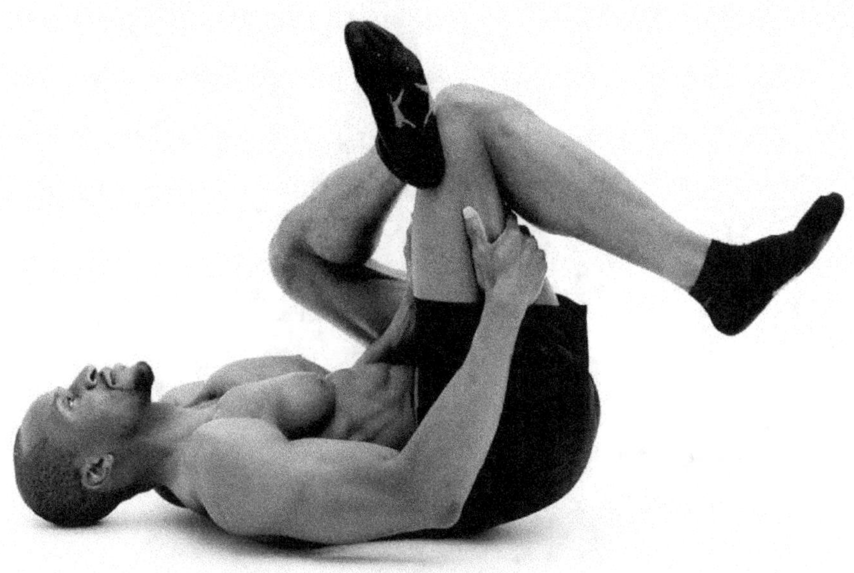

HIP FLEXOR

Your hip flexors work in harmony with your glutes so you can't stretch one without the other. Check this out:

Perform: 30 second hold time on each side

1. Stand upright, then place one foot forward.

2. Bend the knee of your front foot and, keeping your body straight and rear foot on the spot, lean forward.

3. When you feel a stretch in the top of your back leg, hold for allotted time.

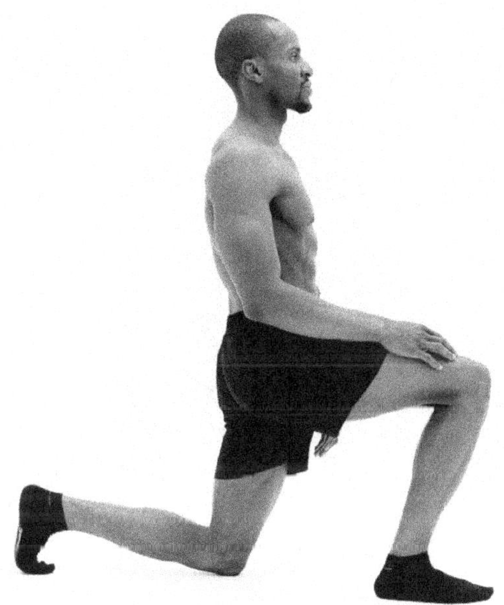

H PS II

Here, we'll focus on your hips, groin, and hammies, areas that are chronically tight in many people.

Perform: 30 second hold.

1. Start at a comfortable sitting position on the floor, and then spread your legs outward as far as you can.

2. Slowly lean forward as far as possible into the space between your legs, and hold for allotted time.

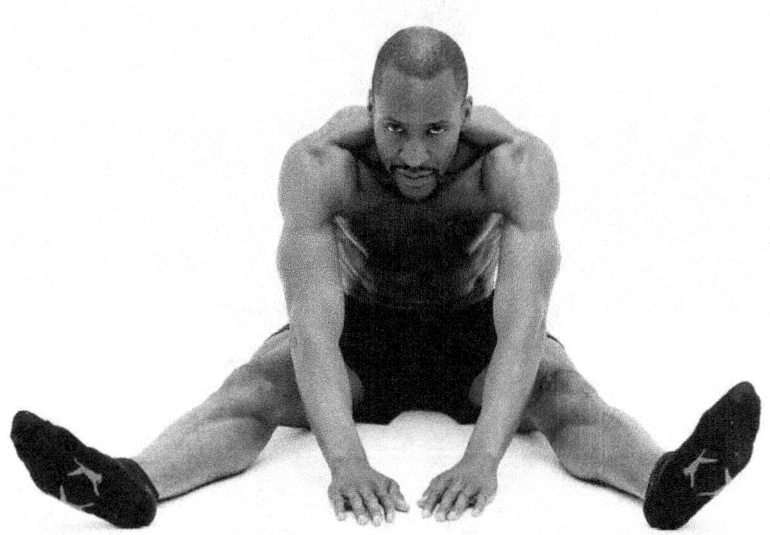

QUADRICEPS

Another massive muscle group vitally important to both calisthenics and day-to-day life are your quads. Keep them happy with this simple stretch:

Perform: 30 second hold time.

1. Lie down flat on your stomach.

2. Bend one knee and bring the foot towards your glutes.

3. Grasp the foot with your hand and pull it towards your glutes, then hold for allotted time.

That covers the essential stretching for major muscle groups. Remember to stretch after each workout to aid recovery and increase range of motion and, subsequently, strength.

Listen to your body and seek advice from a specialist if you are unsure about anything. You should be using this advice as a general guideline to help build your own stretching routine rather than sticking to it exactly as it's written above.

For a comprehensive guide on building superhuman strength through flexibility, pick up our companion book on Amazon. Just search 'Pure Calisthenics Flexibility'.

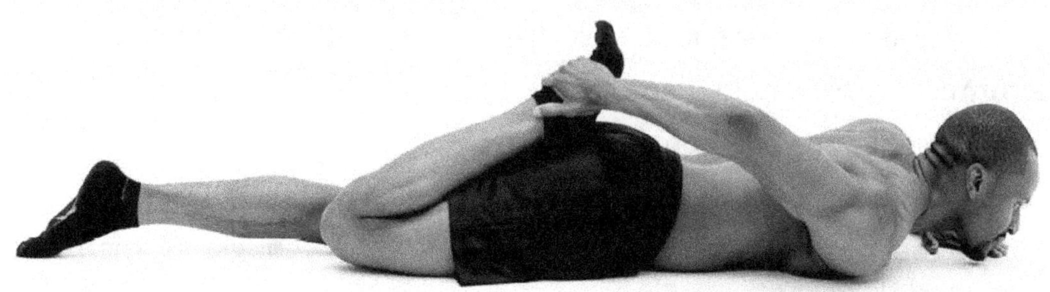

"Take care of your body. It's the only place youhave to live."

Jim Rohn

5. EXERCISES

It's time to get into the good stuff! If you commit to mastering the following exercises and don't throw in the towel when the going gets tough then you WILL experience mind-blowing results.

Disclaimer: This bodyweight training guide has been designed to help you learn the art of calisthenics progressively. Each exercise will start off with the simplest variation, becoming more difficult as you work through the book.

Since we cannot be there to train you in person, we have provided HD photographs and detailed tutorials. We cannot be held accountable for any misuse of instructions or injuries that occur as a result. It is down to you to be smart and attempt only what you are ready for.

Where possible, always use a spotter or personal trainer to ensure you are using the correct form for each exercise. There is no glory or value in squeezing out more sets or reps than someone else if you aren't performing the exercises properly.

Remember: This is a resource created to teach bodyweight exercises, NOT a training program. We cannot suggest an exact amount of sets and reps for you without knowing your level of ability, so the numbers given in this guide are just a suggestion.

If you want to get started with a proper training routine you will find a link at the back of this book to our free companion program. As always, for a more personal approach, hook up with a calisthenics trainer to create a bespoke program.

All that is left to do at this stage is make sure you are sufficiently warmed up before jumping into any of the following exercises. If you skipped the section on warm-up and preparation, do yourself a favor and go back a few steps. It might just be the difference between make or break.

So, you're clued up, you're warmed up, and you're raring to go. Just what kind of crazy exercises are we going to use to achieve SUPERHUMAN form?

Well, the most astonishing thing is, it all starts with the humble push-up.

Let's do this!

UPPER BODY

Ready to build a bulging upper body? It all begins here, so read on and always master the fundamentals before advancing. Don't forget your mobility and flexibility work!

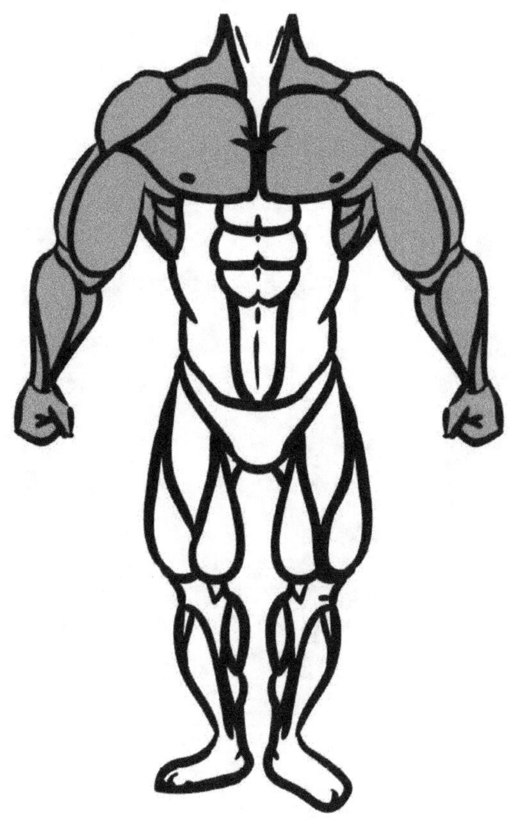

PUSH-UPS

Push-ups are part of our 'essential 12' bodyweight exercises. In fact, they are the very first thing we recommend mastering, since most people already have a grasp on them at some level. Remember not to race ahead to more challenging exercises before you have nailed the basics. If you are attempting things beyond your capabilities your form will suffer and you will do more harm to your body than good. With that said, let's go!

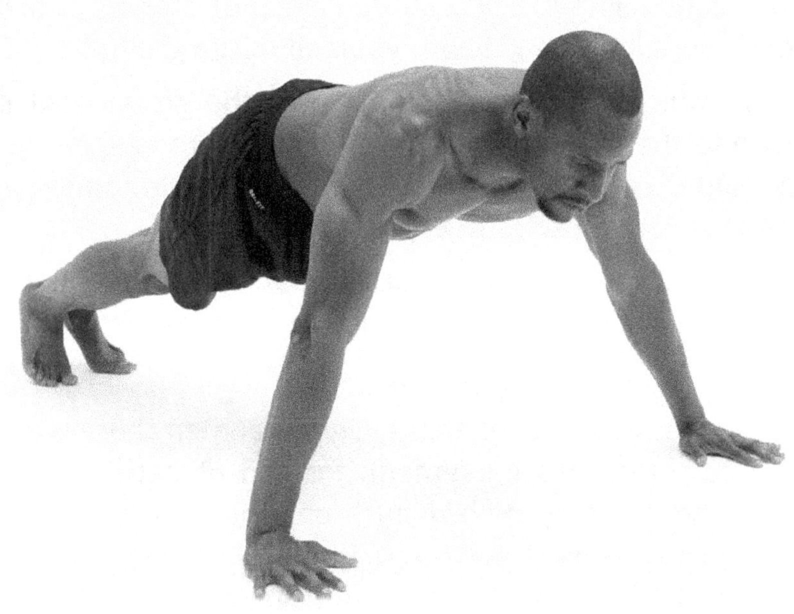

STANDARD PUSH-UP

This is one of the pillars of calisthenics, and it is essential learn it with the proper form. Check it out here and see if you can complete the allocated sets and reps.

Perform: 3-4 sets of 8-12 repetitions (reps).

1. Place your palms flat on the floor, shoulder width apart.

2. Push up onto your hands and toes, keeping your feet close together and your legs, hips and shoulders in a straight line.

3. With your chin slightly raised so you are not staring straight at the ground, bend your elbows and lower yourself to the ground.

4. Stop when your chest makes contact with the ground but do not lie down or drop to the floor completely. Remember to keep your body in a straight line and do not let your stomach touch the ground – you should be engaging your core muscles to prevent this.

5. Push yourself back up hard, ensuring your body remains locked in a straight line. You have now completed one repetition!

Variations:

If you are new to push-ups or exercise in general then there is no shame in struggling to complete this movement. Instead of battling through with bad form, try the platform or box push-ups for an easier alternative as shown next. Once you have mastered 3 sets of 10 reps with the proper form, go back and try the standard push-up again.

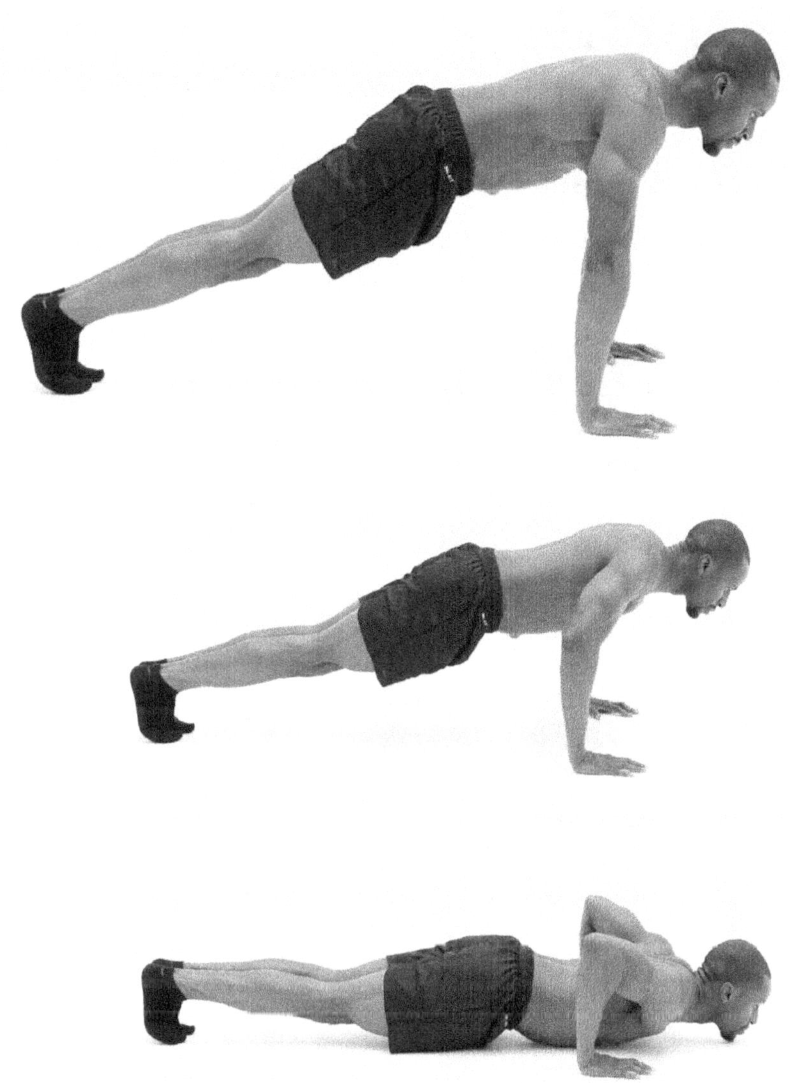

Box PUSH-UP

Not to be confused with the platform push-up (next), this is the easiest version of the movement.

Perform: 3-4 sets of 8-12 repetitions (reps).

1. Get onto your hands and knees, keeping your feet close together.

2. Bend your elbows and lower yourself to the ground.

3. Stop when your head gets close to the ground. You can increase the angle and make things more difficult by bringing your knees back further.

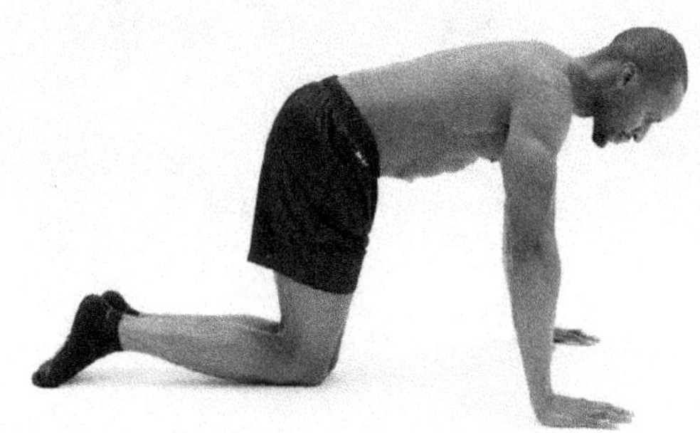

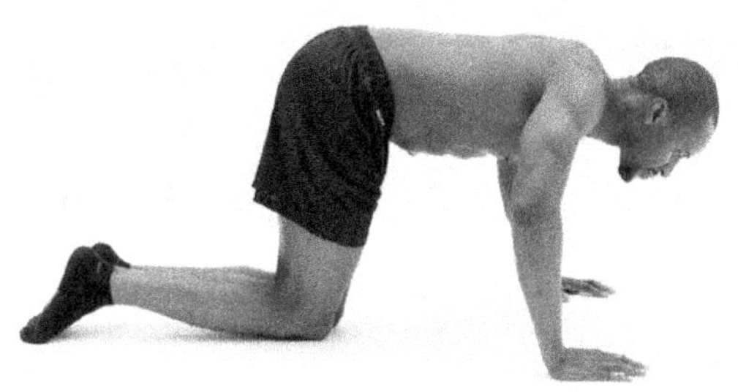

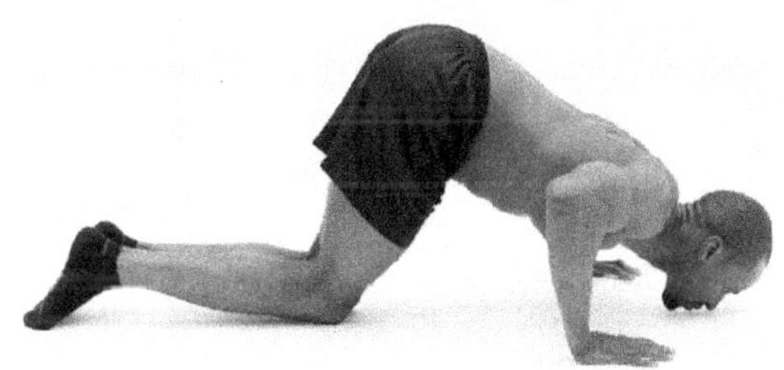

PLATFORM INCLINE PUSH-UP

You can use any raised surface to perform this version. It's perfect if you are struggling with form or simply want to switch up your technique.

Perform: 3-4 sets of 8-12 repetitions (reps).

You will need: a sturdy platform.

1. Place your feet on the floor and your hands on a sturdy platform.

2. Bend your elbows and lower yourself towards the platform.

3. Stop when your chest reaches the platform. Note that the higher it is, the easier this variation will be.

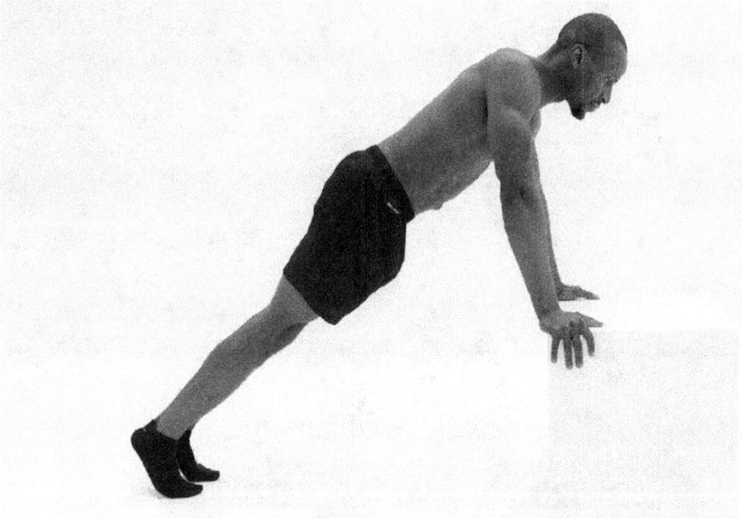

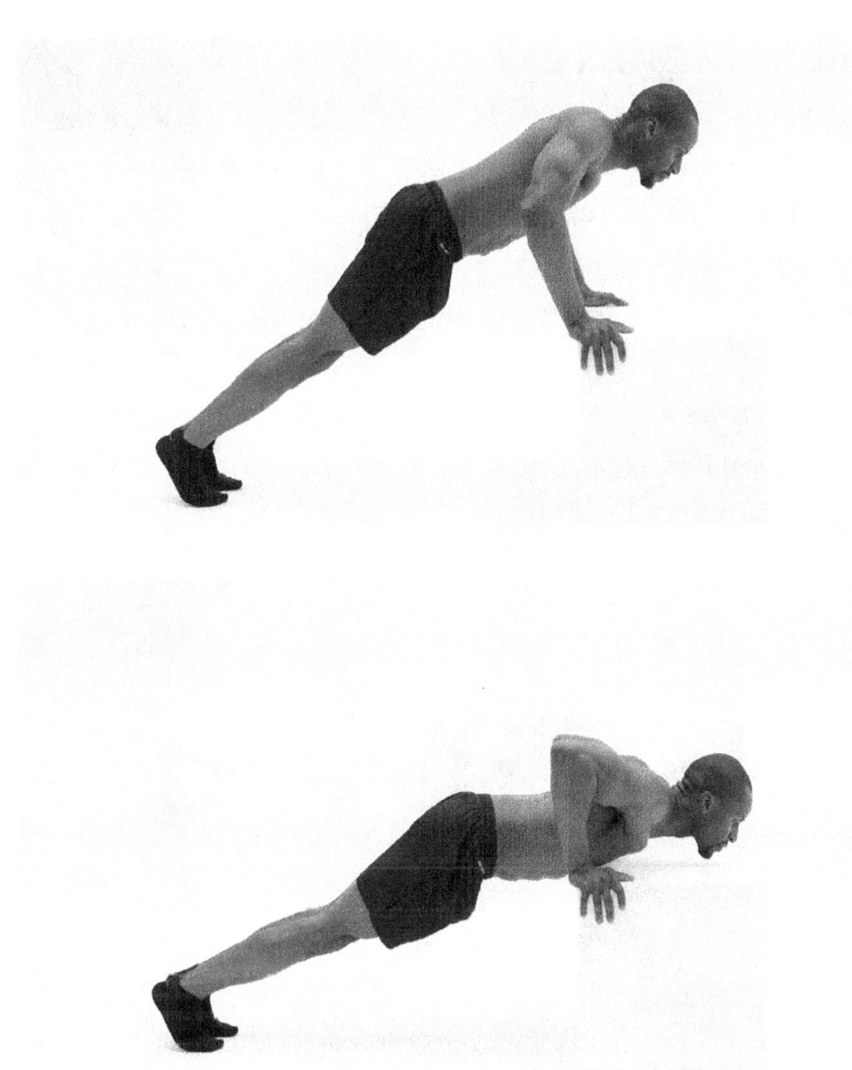

PLATFORM DECLINE PUSH-UP

Swap your hands and feet around on the platform to increase the challenge and send your chest and shoulders into overdrive!

Perform: 3-4 sets of 8-12 repetitions (reps).

You will need: a sturdy platform.

1. Place your feet on the platform and your hands on the floor in front of you.

2. Bend your elbows and lower yourself towards the platform.

3. Stop when your chest reaches the platform. Note that the higher the platform is, the more difficult this will become.

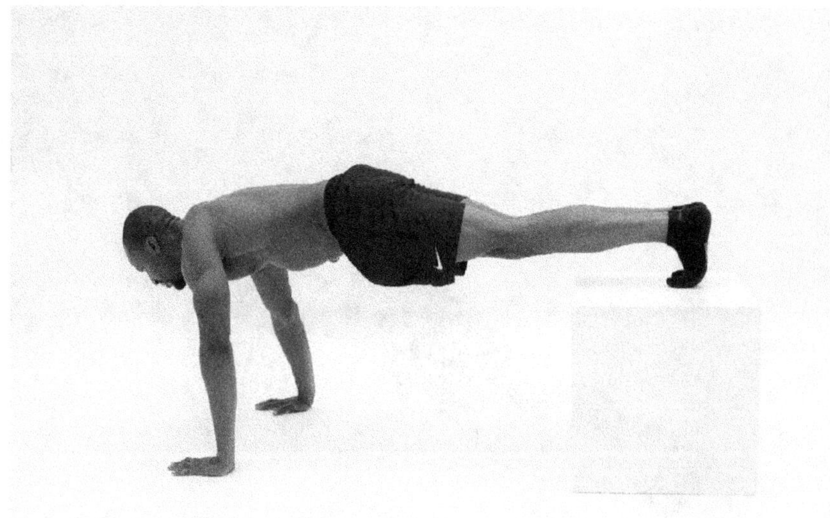

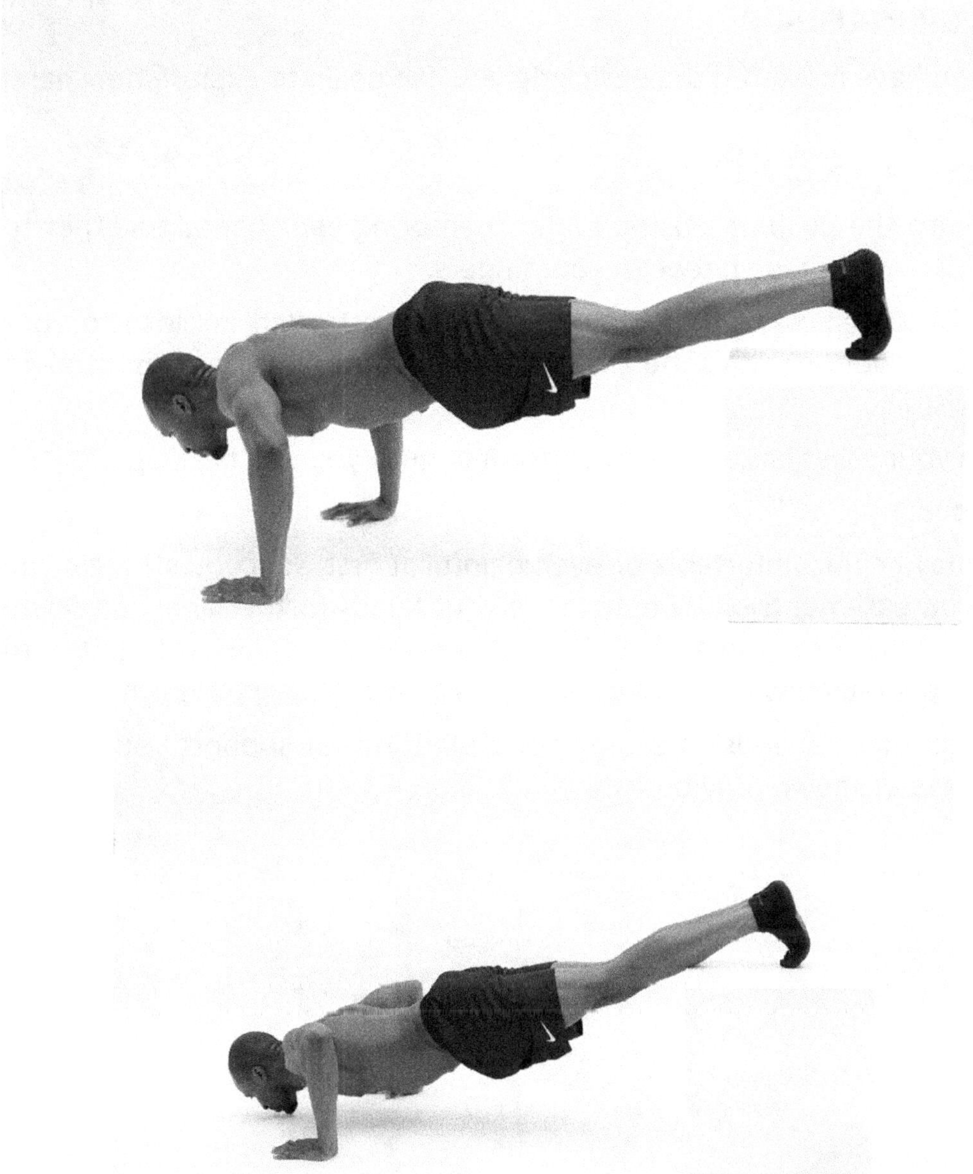

CLOSE GRIP PUSH-UP

Once you have mastered the basic grip you can begin to explore new hand positions.

Perform: 3-4 sets of 8-12 reps.

1. Get into the push-up position, and then bring your hands together to form a diamond shape between your fingers.

2. Bend your elbows and, keeping your elbows tucked in close to your sides, lower your chest to the ground ensuring your body remains straight as always.

3. Once your chest has touched the ground, push yourself back up.

Variations:

• This may be uncomfortable or even painful at first, so if you struggle you can try an easier version. Simply move your hands further apart until you are able to perform 3 sets of 10 reps. Move your hands closer together to increase the difficulty over time.

• Another alternative is to use a raised platform, or support yourself on your knees as shown previously.

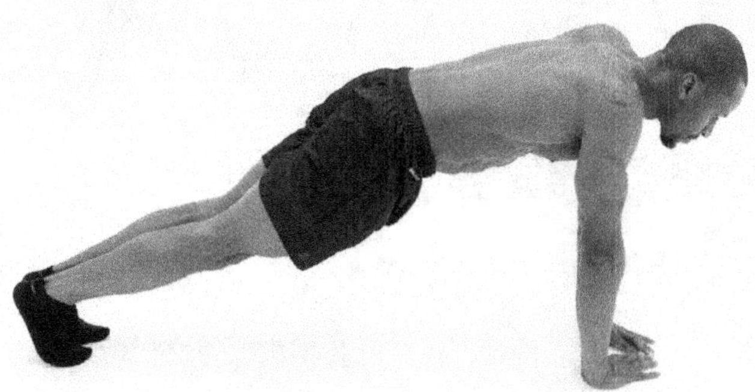

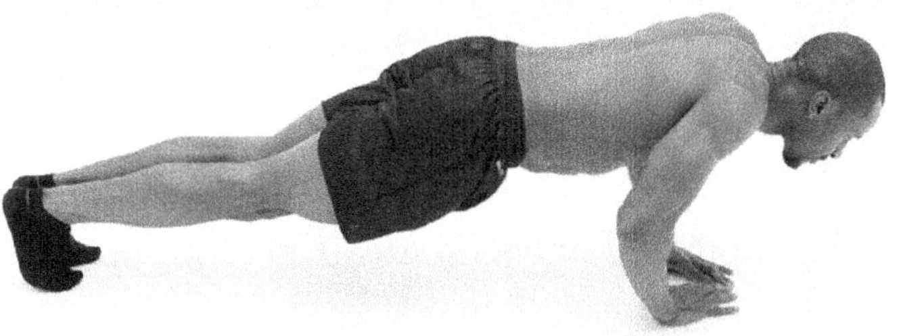

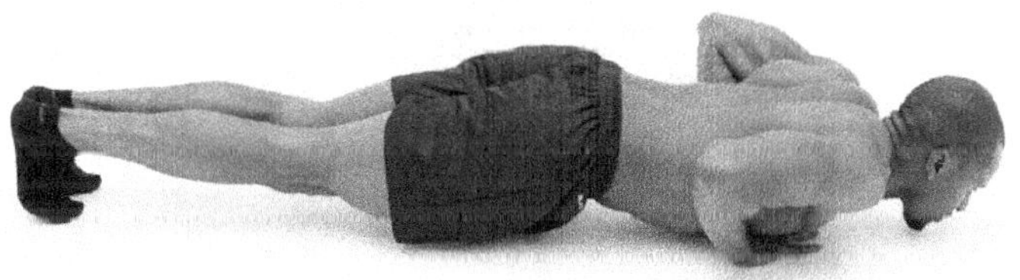

WIDE GRIP PUSH-UP

This is another variation on the standard push-up. Combining this with the previous two gives you a great basis for a ripped chest arm bulging arms!

Perform: 3-4 sets of 8-12 reps.

1. Get into standard push-up position, then place your hands as wide apart as possible ensuring your chest stays off the ground and your shoulders, hips and legs remain in a straight line.

2. Bend your elbows and lower your chest to the ground.

3. Push yourself back up to the starting position to complete a rep.

Variations:

• If you find this too difficult, try moving your hands inwards a little until you reach a point where you can complete the allotted reps. Over time you will be able to progress to a wider grip.

• The variations shown in the standard push-up are also an option here.

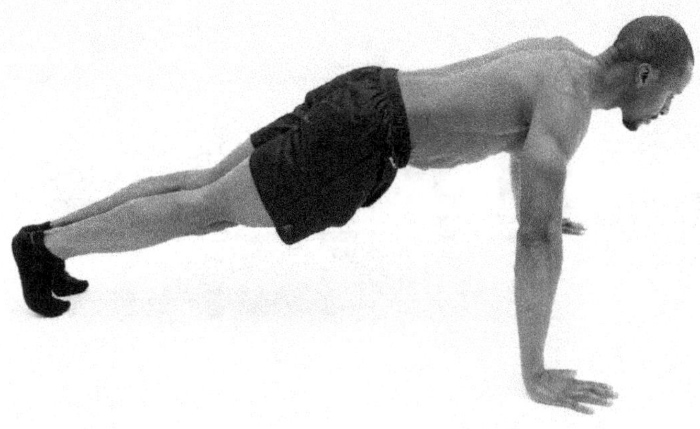

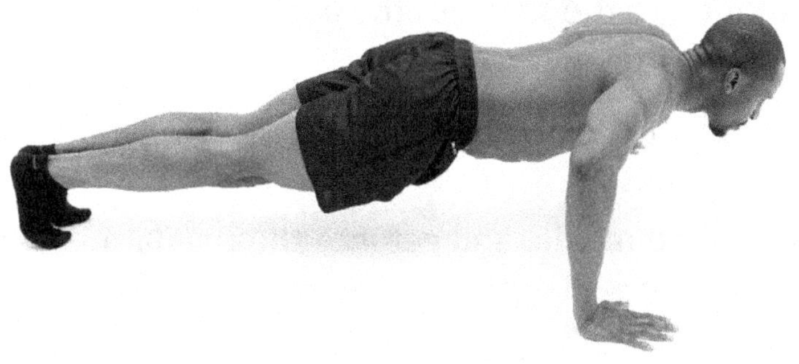

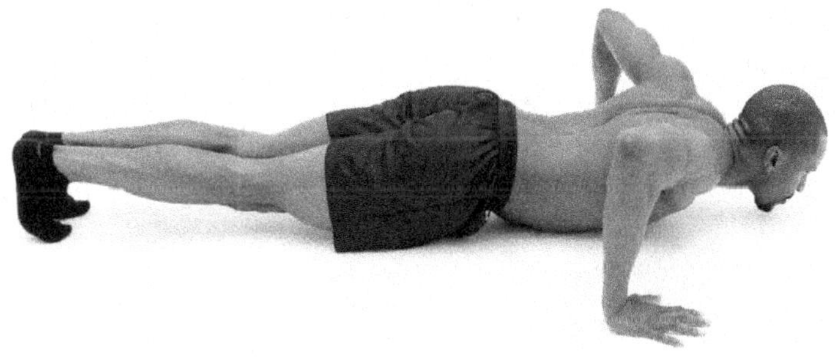

DEEP PUSH-UP

Designed to push you to your limits, this will yield phenomenal results when done with the proper form. Though this is primarily a chest and arm exercise, pay attention to the shape of the back also.

Perform: 3-4 sets of 8-12 reps.

You will need: parallettes or two strong and secure parallel bars such as dumbbells with a flat bottom.

1. Grab both bars in the middle and get into the regular push-up position, making sure the bars are well rooted and sturdy.

2. Ensuring your body remains in a straight line as always, bend your elbows and slowly lower your chest downwards as far as you can comfortably go.

3. When you reach your maximum depth, push yourself back up again and to complete a rep, then repeat the process.

Beginners may not be able to get their chest to dip below their elbows. Don't force it as this may result in injury. Instead, practice this exercise regularly and you will gradually increase your range of motion. Your warm-up and preparation will also be a factor here.

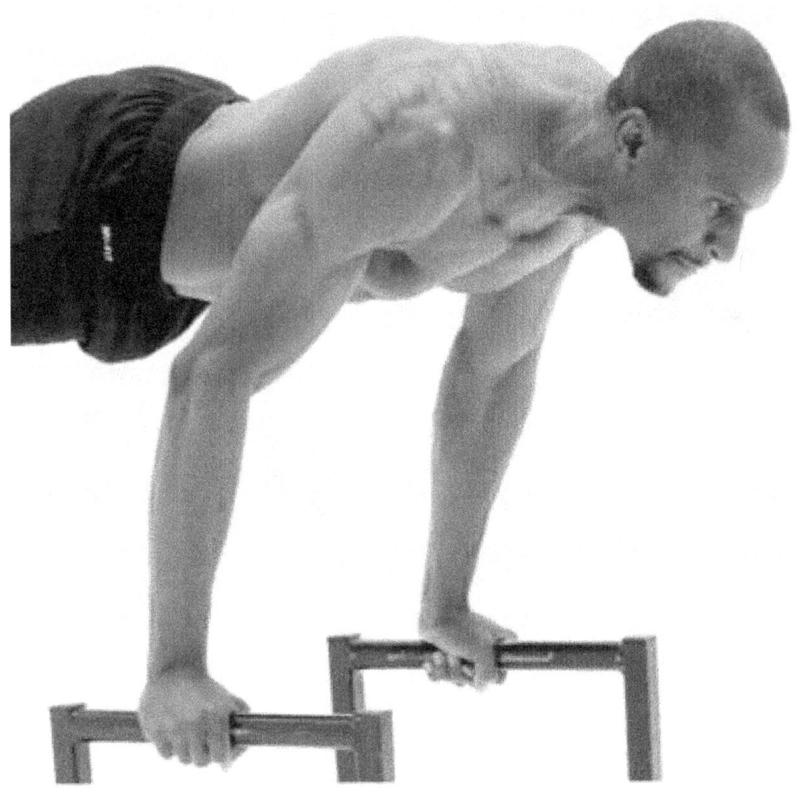

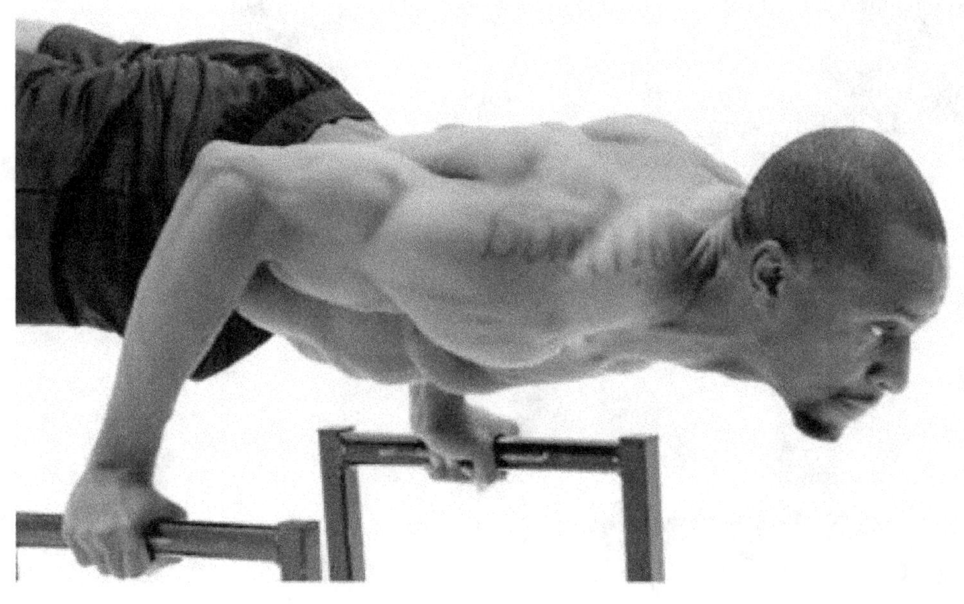

"The vision of a champion is bent over, drenched in sweat, at the point of exhaustion, when nobody else is looking."

Mia Hamm

D PS

Dips are another exercise in the 'pushing' family and are particularly good for targeting the triceps, chest and shoulders. This is another staple exercise to add to your arsenal!

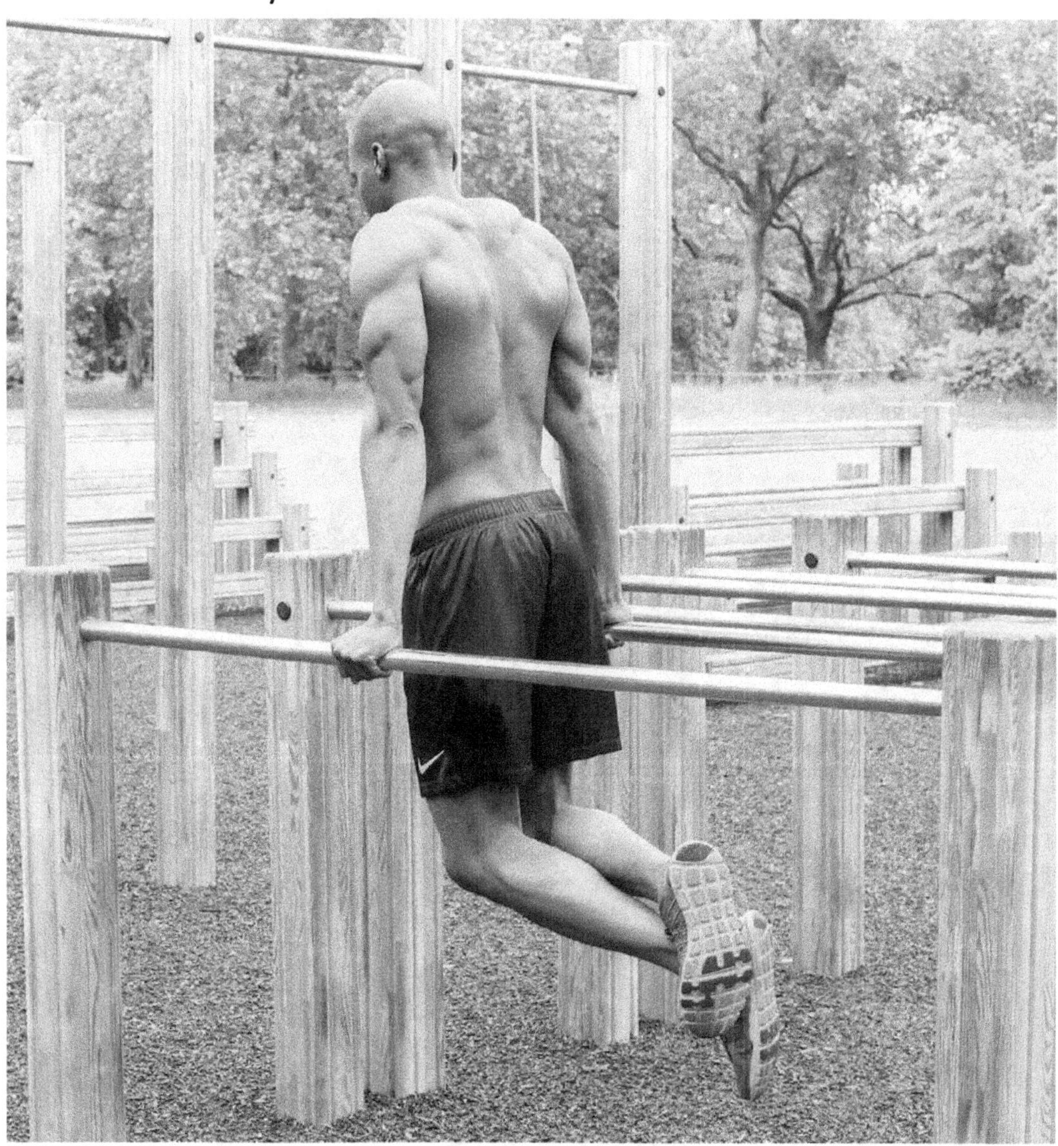

PLATFORM DIPS

This little number will get your triceps pumped and prepare you for the full version next.

Perform: 3-4 sets of 8-12 reps.

You will need: a box or sturdy raised platform.

1. With your back to the platform, place your palms on the edge and allow your fingers to rest on the front, securing your grip.

2. Stretch both legs straight out in front of you with your knees locked and rest on your heels.

3. Bend your elbows and lower yourself to the ground, keeping your back as straight and close to the platform as possible.

4. When your reach your maximum depth, push yourself back up again to complete the first rep.

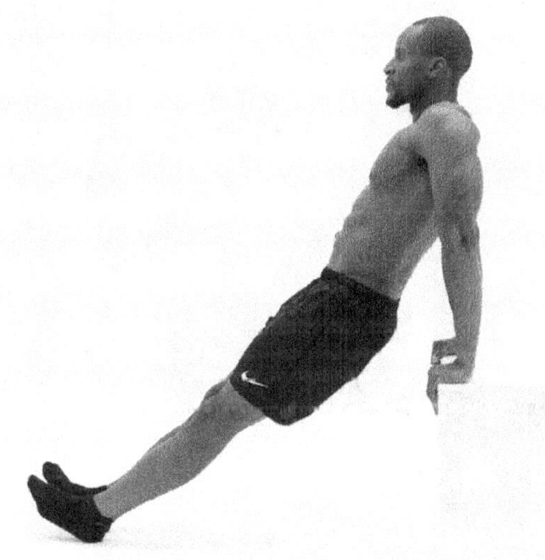

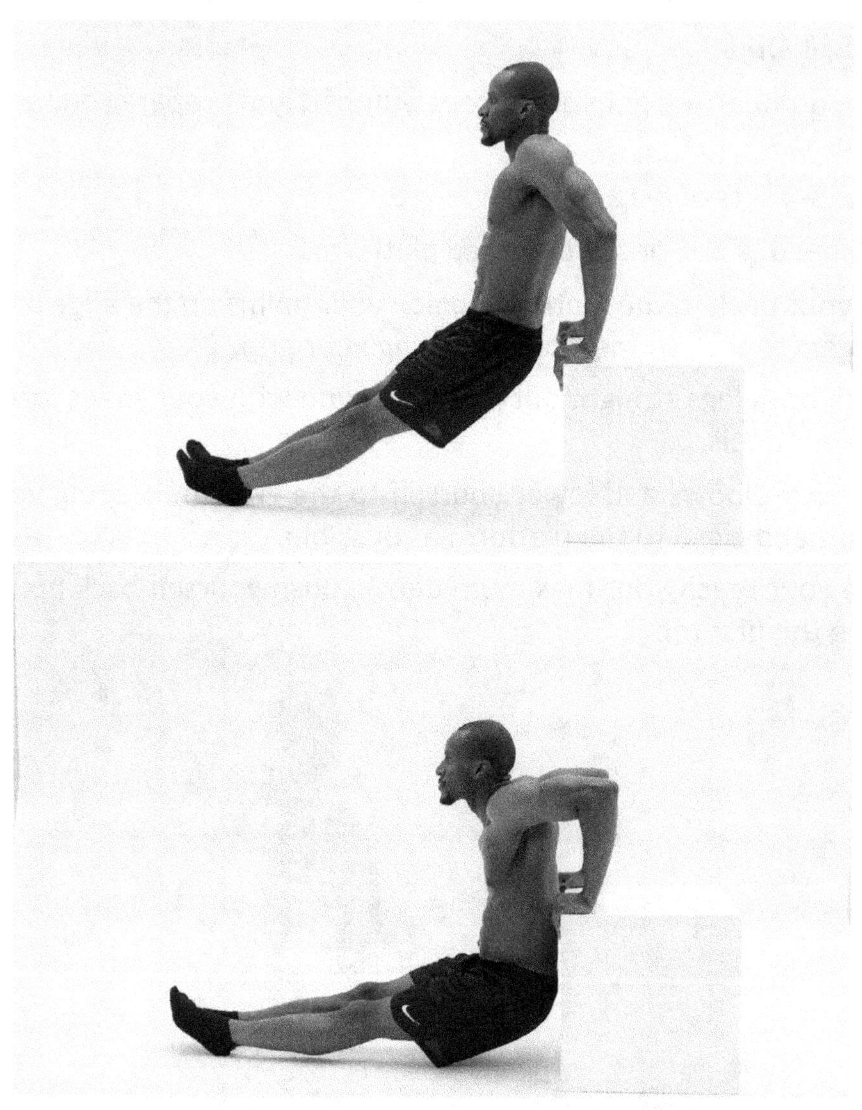

PARALLEL BAR DIPS

By lifting your feet up off the floor your are now supporting your entire bodyweight. This exercise will be tougher than the last, so remember to focus on your form and go back a step if you are finding it too difficult.

Perform: 3-4 sets of 8-12 reps.

You will need: dip station.

1. Grab the bars with your palms facing in towards your body. If your feet are touching the ground, lock them together and raise them behind you at a 90-degree angle.

2. Bend your elbows and lower yourself down as far as possible.

3. When you reach your maximum depth, push back up again and lock your elbows to complete the first rep.

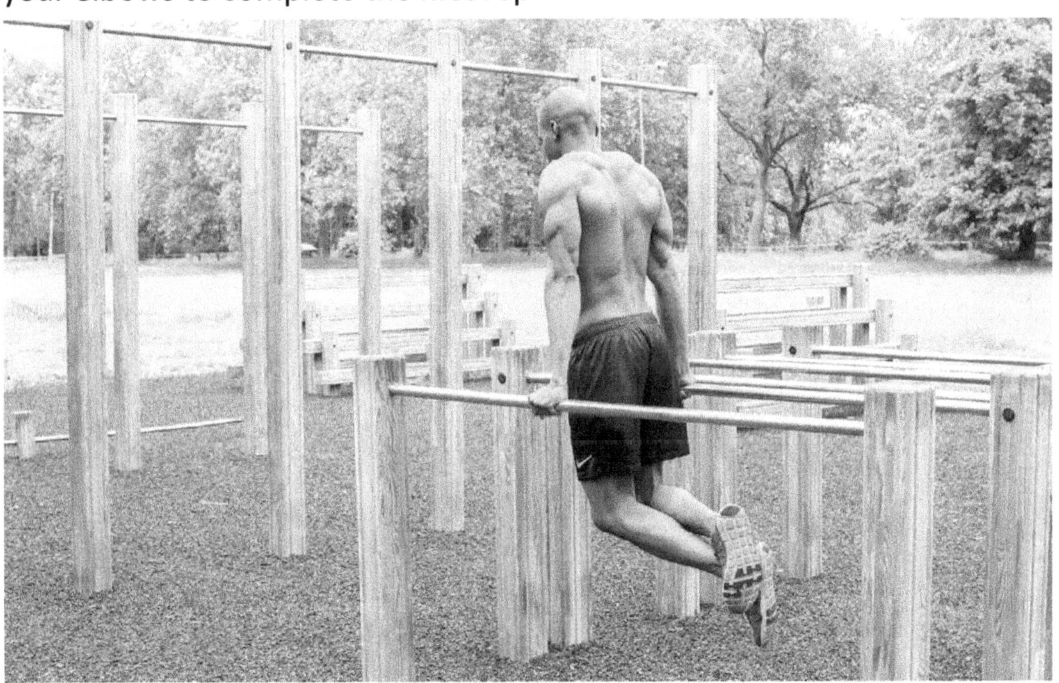

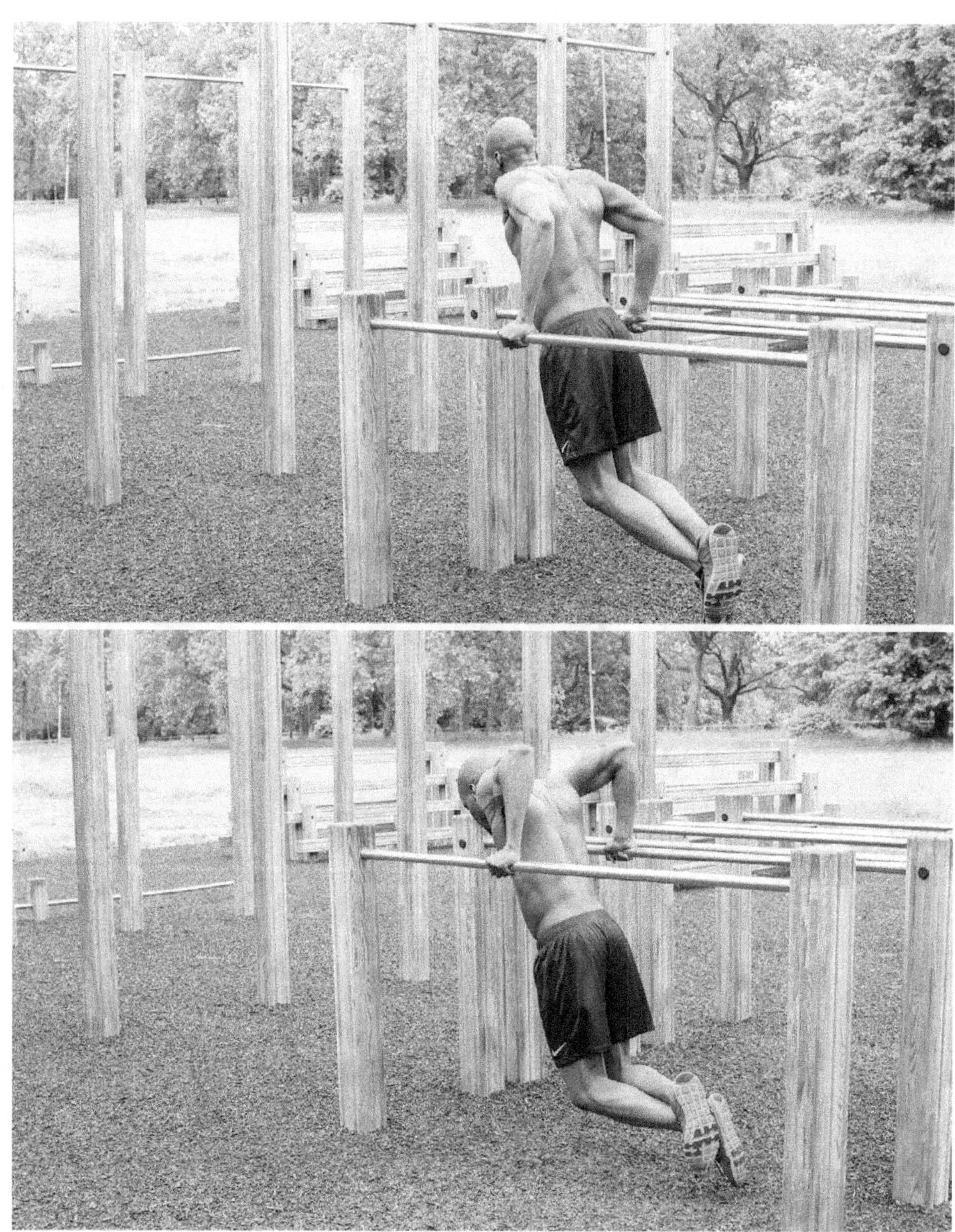

STRAIGHT BAR DIPS

This is the most difficult dip movement, so take your time and make sure you are using proper form. You might find it useful to have a spotter take some of the weight off when first training for this exercise, as it is brutally taxing on your upper body and core.

Perform: 3-4 sets of 8-12 reps.

You will need: a straight, secure bar.

1. Grab the bar with your palms facing down and hands shoulder width apart.

2. Making sure there is nothing above to bang your head on, raise yourself up until your elbows lock. This is starting position.

3. Bend your elbows and lower your body downwards. If your body / legs naturally go forwards to aid with balance, that is fine.

4. When you get as low as possible, push yourself back up until your elbows lock again to complete one rep.

NB: This exercise is a great foundation for the muscle-up, an immensely challenging exercise which combines pulling and pushing on the bar.

The muscle-up is a favorite among the calisthenics community, so it pays to train with straight bar dips in order to establish a firm foundation.

Likewise, if you find yourself struggling with the muscle-up later on, switch back to the straight bar dip to top up your pushing power.

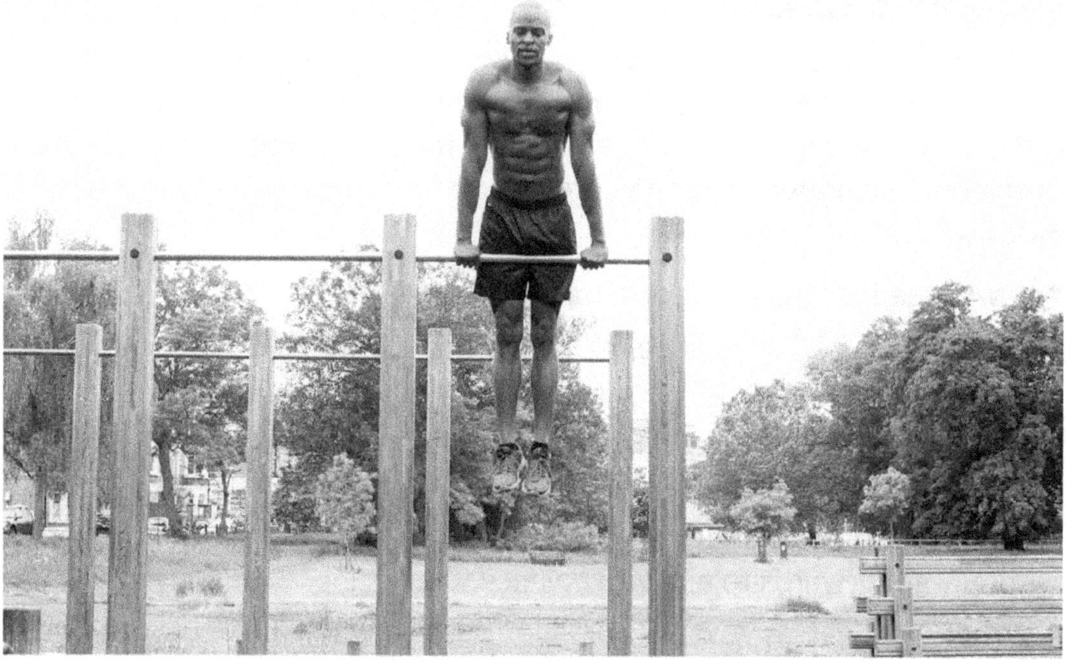

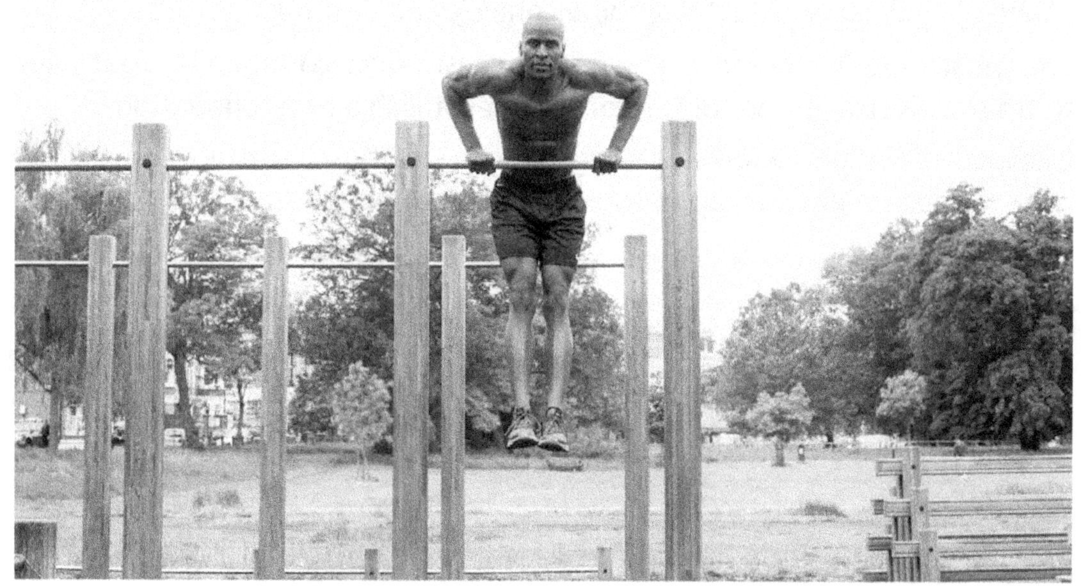

PULL-UPS / CHIN-UPS

Now that we've covered the key pushing exercises we can move on to pulling in order to target different muscle groups. Pull-ups are a complete upper body exercise that are especially good for targeting the muscles in your arms and back. Prepare for progress!

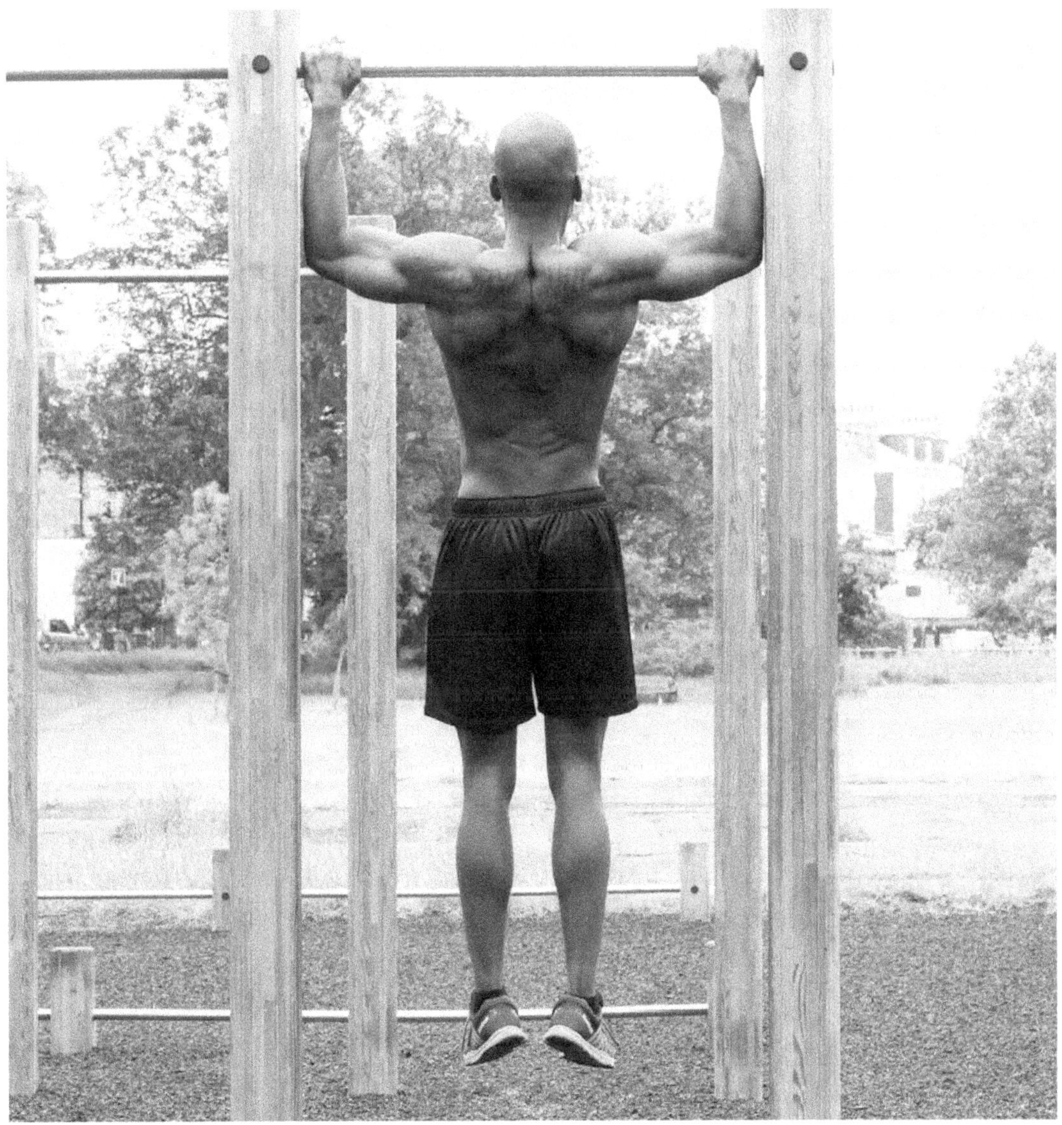

RAISED BAR Row

This is a good place to start if you are completely new to pull-ups as, similar to raised platform push-ups, the more favorable angle makes the exercise easier to complete.

Perform: 3-4 sets of 8-12 reps.

You will need: a sturdy and secure bar.

1. Grab the bar with an overhand grip and straighten your arms.

2. Walk your legs forward in front of the bar so your body is at an angle (the greater the angle, the more difficult the exercise.) This is start position.

3. Ensuring your body stays straight and your feet remain in position, pull your chest up until it touches the bar.

4. When your chest has touched the bar or gone as far as possible, lower yourself back down and straighten your arms to complete one rep.

Variations:

• Move the bar up to make the exercise easier, or down to make it harder.

• Use TRX straps instead of a bar.

• Use an underhand grip.

• Move your hands closer / further apart.

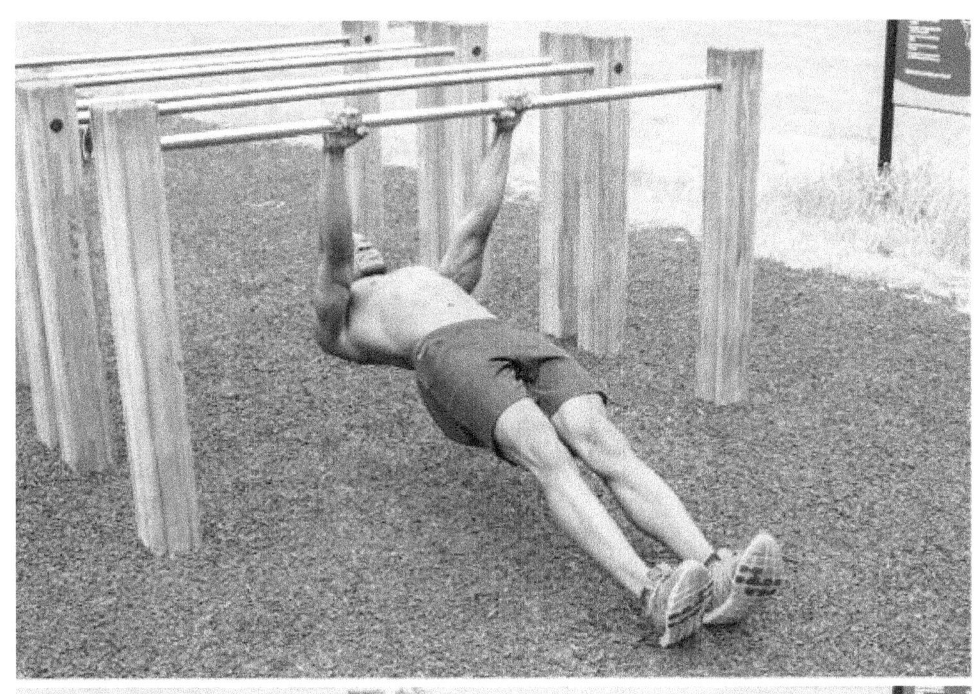

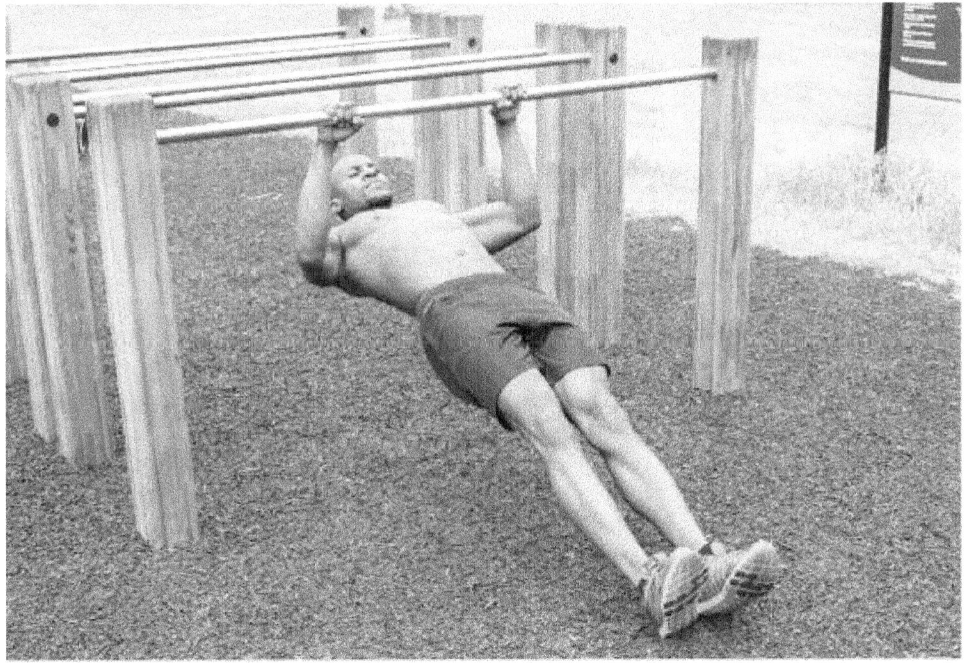

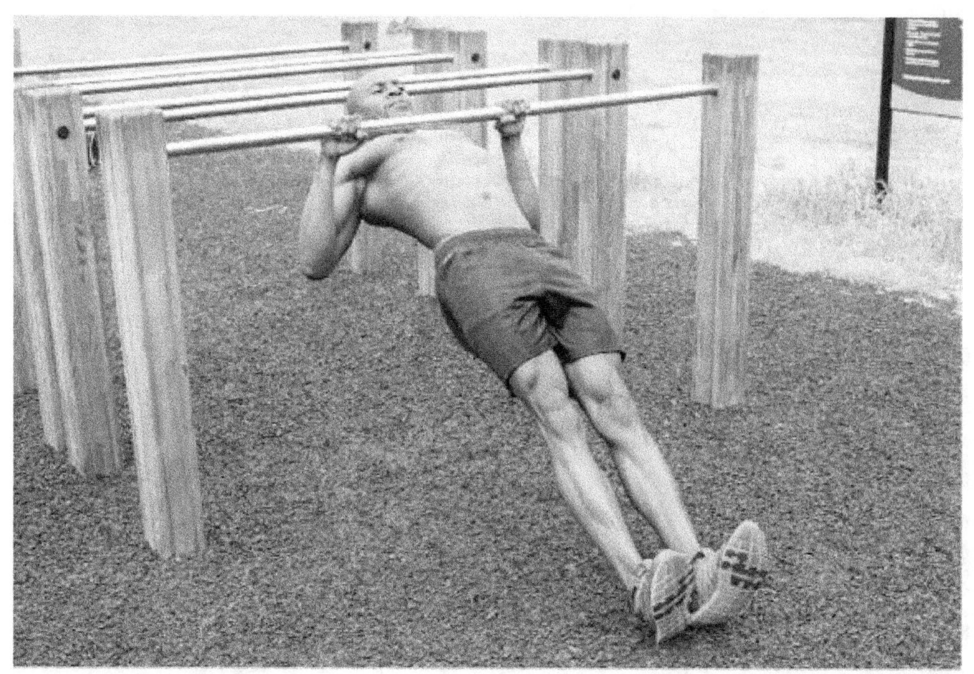

NEGATIVE CHIN-UP

Chin-ups can be an intimidating exercise to master but fortunately, as with most other calisthenics exercises, there is a simpler variation you can try first.

Perform: 3-4 sets of 3-5 reps.

You will need: a pull-up bar.

1. Get to the top position of a chin-up, using a platform, spotter or simply jumping if you can't quite make it under your own steam.

2. Slowly lower yourself down, tensing your muscles to work them as much as possible, until your arms are straight and elbows are locked, then drop off the bar to complete one rep and reset.

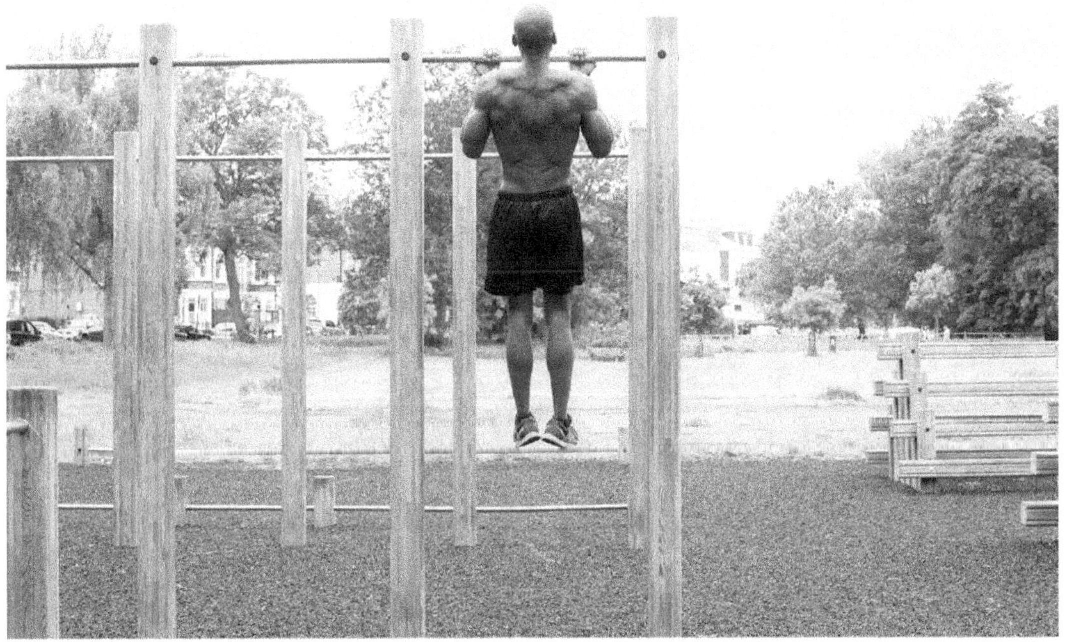

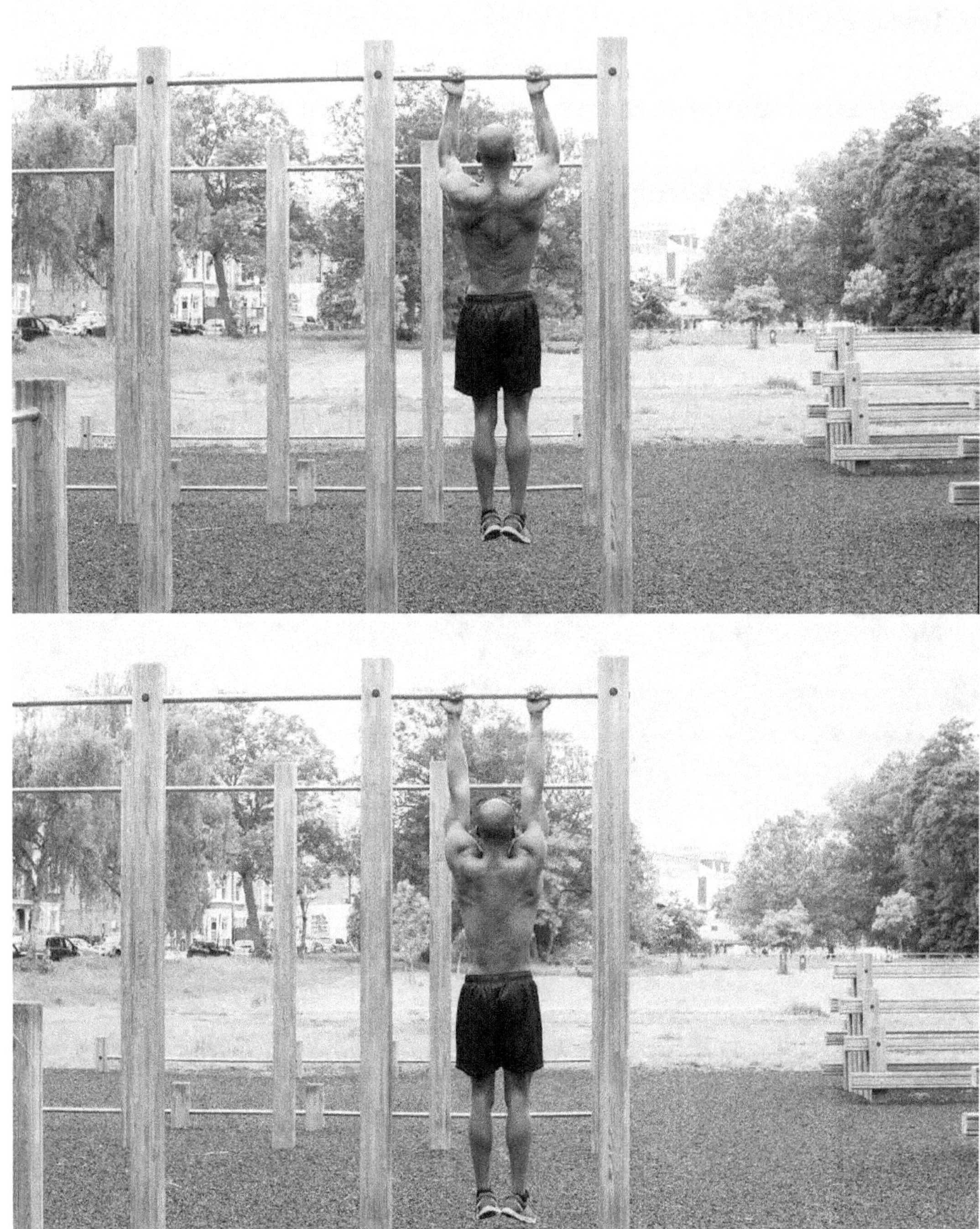

STATIC HOLD

Another simple variation on the pull-up is one that requires no movement at all in order to build the strength required to dive into the full version.

Perform: 20 second hold time.

You will need: a pull-up bar.

1. Achieve the position you wish to hold by pulling, jumping, using a box or lowering yourself into it.

2. Lock your muscles in place and try to hold this position for the allotted time.

3. Once complete, slowly lower yourself down and drop off the bar. If you don't quite complete the allotted time, throw in as many sets as it takes to reach that total amount e.g. 2x 10 seconds = 20 seconds.

NB: This differs from the negative chin-up in that you will be spending as much time as possible holding your position to build strength and endurance.

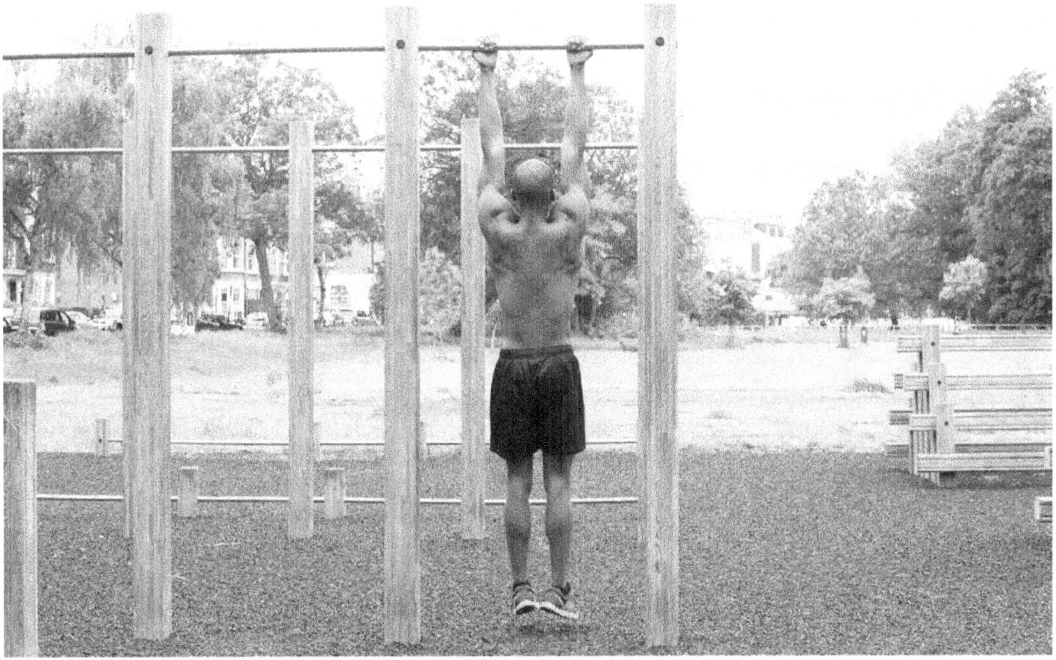

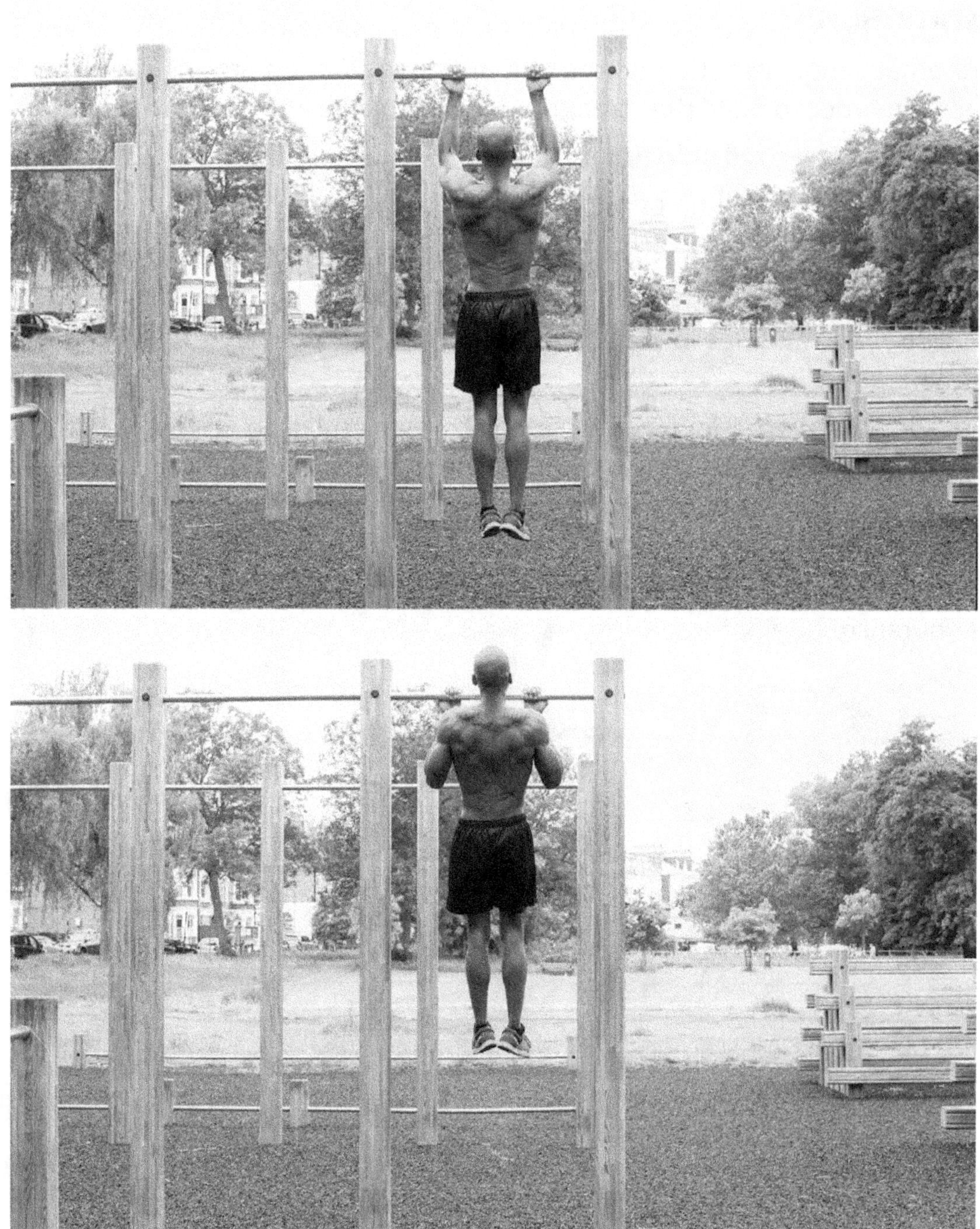

CHIN-UP

Once you can comfortably perform the introductory exercises you can move onto the real thing! Chin-ups are the easiest of the full bodyweight pulling exercises as they leverage the two muscle groups that tend to already be strongest; the biceps and chest.

That said this can still be difficult for beginners so remember to focus on your form and go with quality over quantity!

Perform: 3-4 sets of 8-12 reps.

You will need: a pull-up bar.

1. Using an underhand grip, grab the bar with your hands approximately shoulder width apart.

2. Relax your shoulders, allowing them to sag down. Lock your elbows and lift your feet up so you are hanging freely. This is your starting position.

3. Pull your body up as high as possible, the aim being to get your chin above the bar or have your chest touch against it. Do not swing your body or legs or use momentum to help you.

4. When you reach the top position, lower yourself back down slowly and hang freely again to complete the first rep.

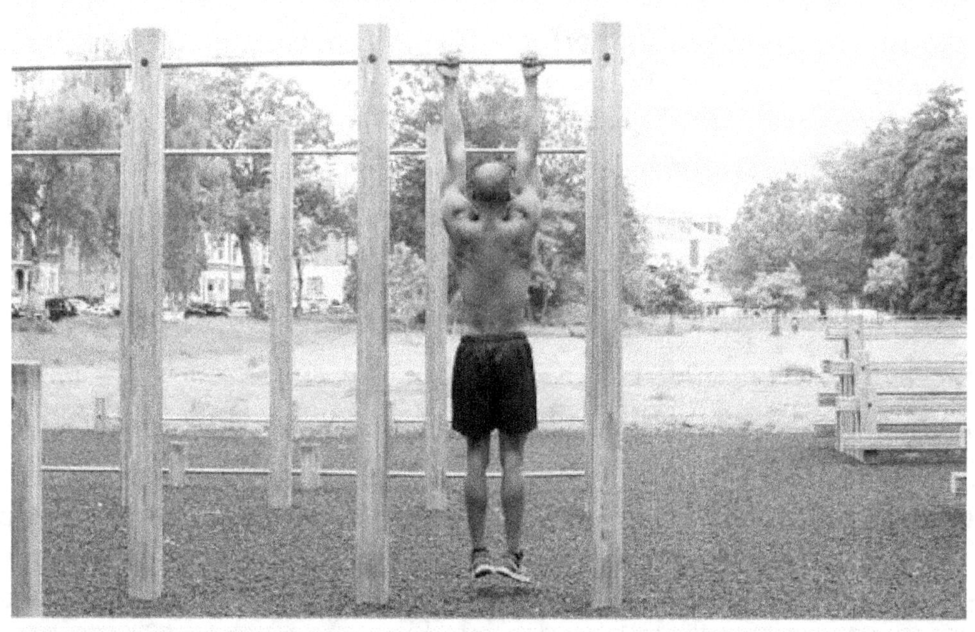

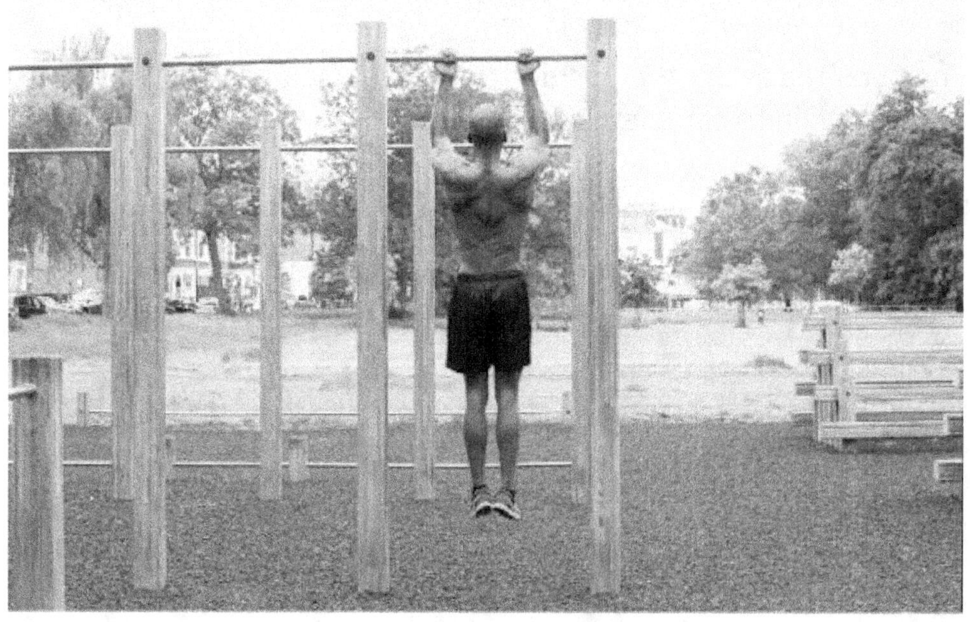

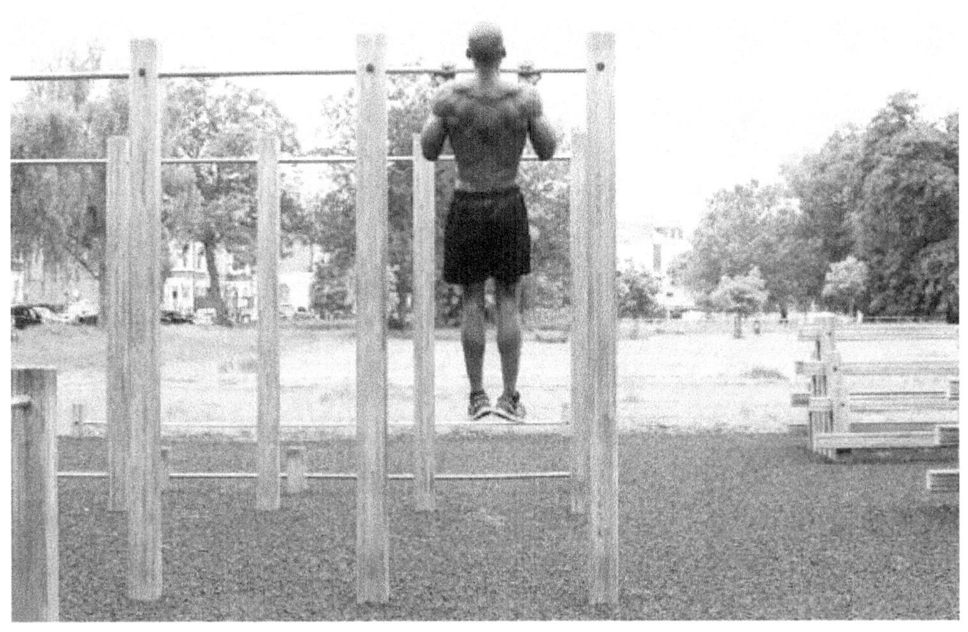

P---- U

This exercise essentially follows the same formula as the chin-up, but with one crucial difference; overhand instead of underhand grip.

By changing to this grip you are taking away much of the biceps' ability to assist with the lift, effectively transferring that effort and energy to your back, specifically the lats.

Again, feel free to perform rows, negatives and statics in order to build your way up to this exercise.

Perform: 3-4 sets of 8-12 reps.

You will need: a pull-up bar.

1. Grab the pull-up bar using an overhand grip with your hands approximately shoulder width apart.

2. Lift your feet off the ground and hang with your elbows locked straight to achieve start position.

3. Keeping your legs and body straight and without using momentum, pull yourself up towards the bar until your chin is above it or your chest is touching it.

4. From here, lower yourself down to the start position to complete one rep.

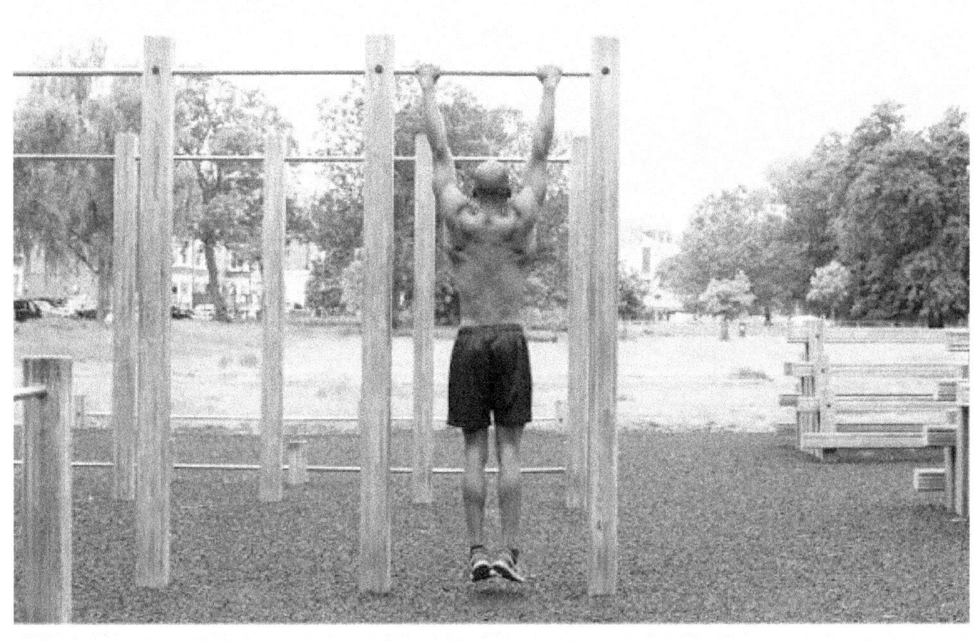

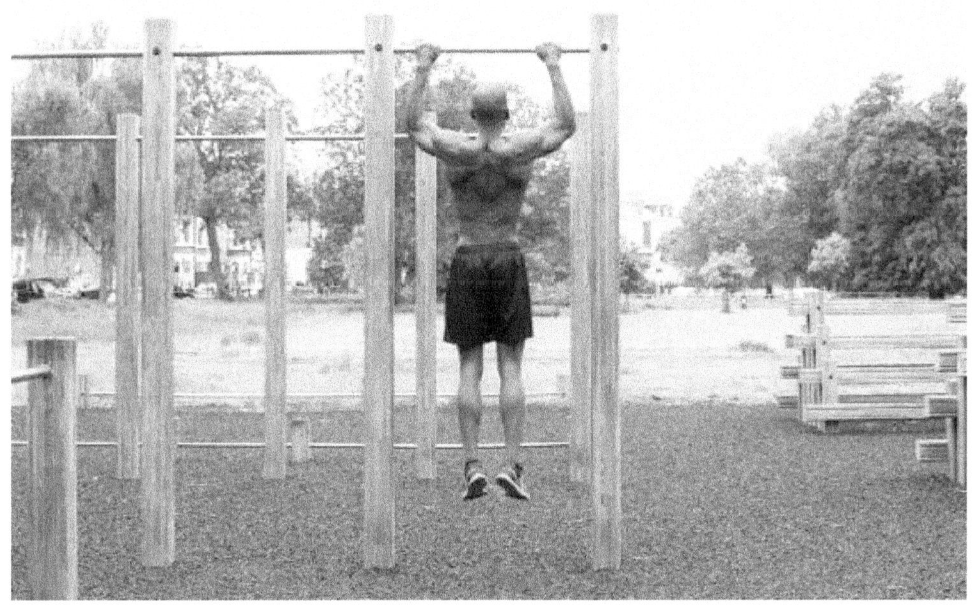

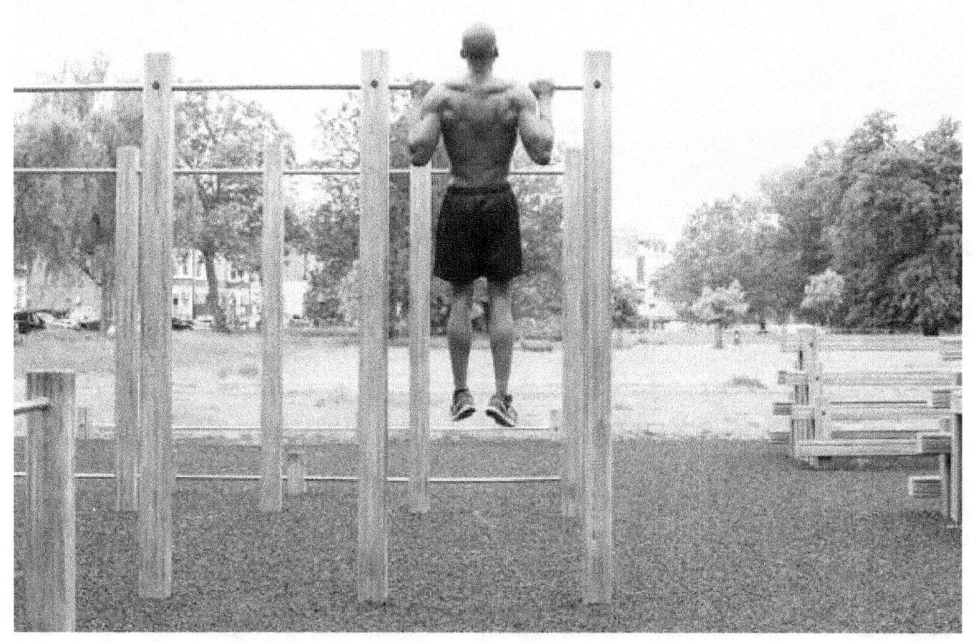

CLOSE GRIP PULL-UP

This is a simple variation on the pull-up that will bring variety to your upper body workout by targeting slightly different areas of the arms and back.

Perform: 3-4 sets of 8-12 reps.

You will need: a pull-up bar.

1. Grab the pull-up bar using an overhand grip with your hands close together.

2. Lift your feet off the ground and hang with your elbows locked straight. You're ready to get started now.

3. Keeping your legs and body straight and without using momentum, pull yourself up towards the bar until your chin is above it or your chest is touching it.

4. From here, lower yourself down to the start position to complete one rep.

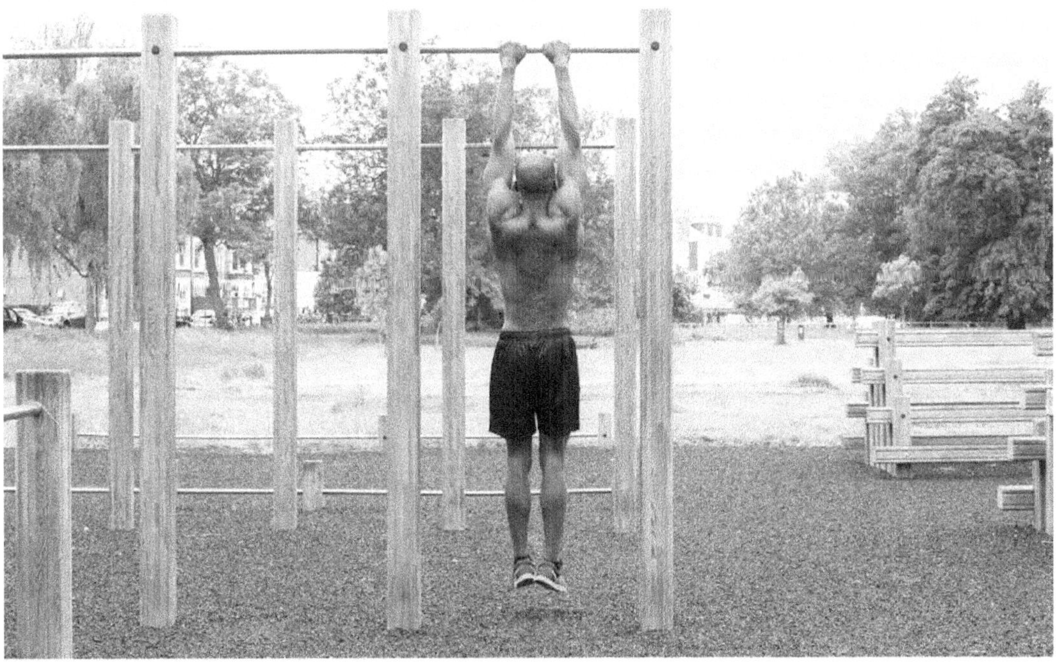

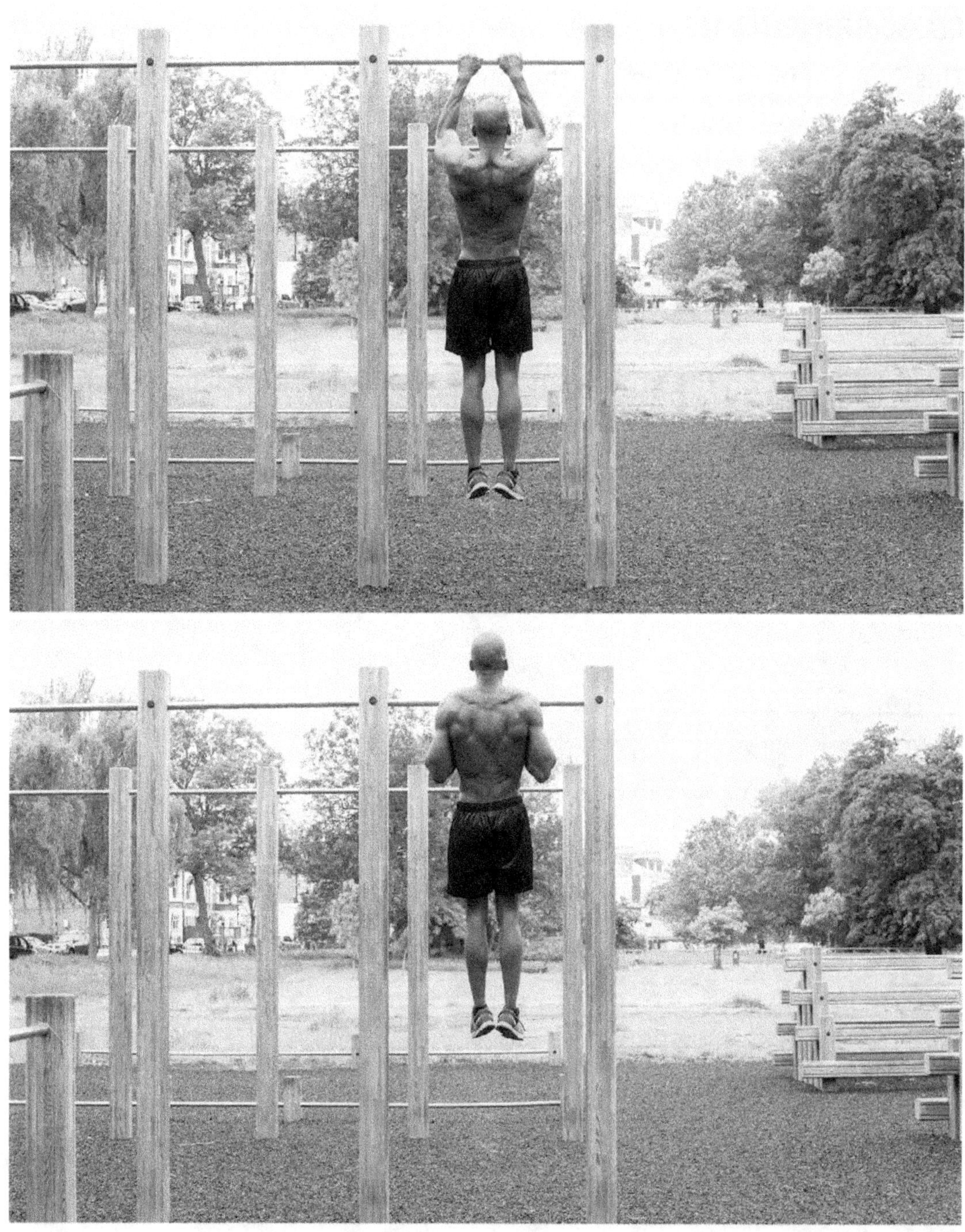

WIDE GRIP PULL-UP

Effectively the opposite of the previous exercise, this is one that will really test your back strength. Both can also be done in chin-up form.

Perform: 3-4 sets of 8-12 reps.

You will need: a pull-up bar.

1. Grab the pull-up bar using an overhand grip with your hands close together.

2. As you now know, lift your feet off the ground and hang with your elbows locked straight to get into the starting position.

3. Keeping your legs and body straight and without using momentum, pull yourself up towards the bar until your chin is above it or your chest is touching it.

4. Lower down to the start position to complete one rep. Go straight into the next rep.

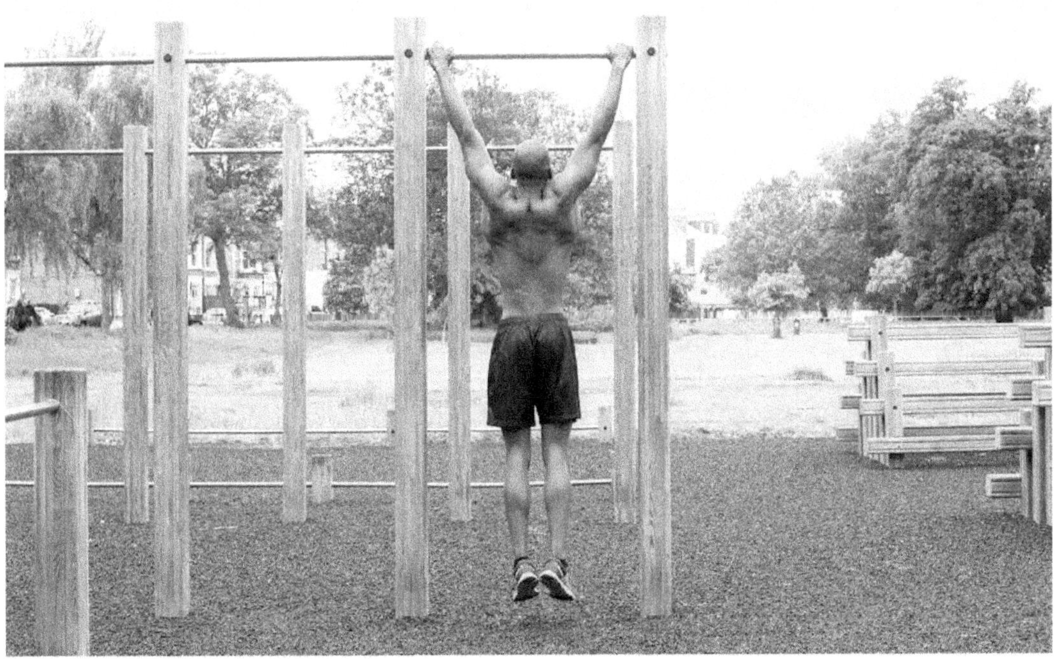

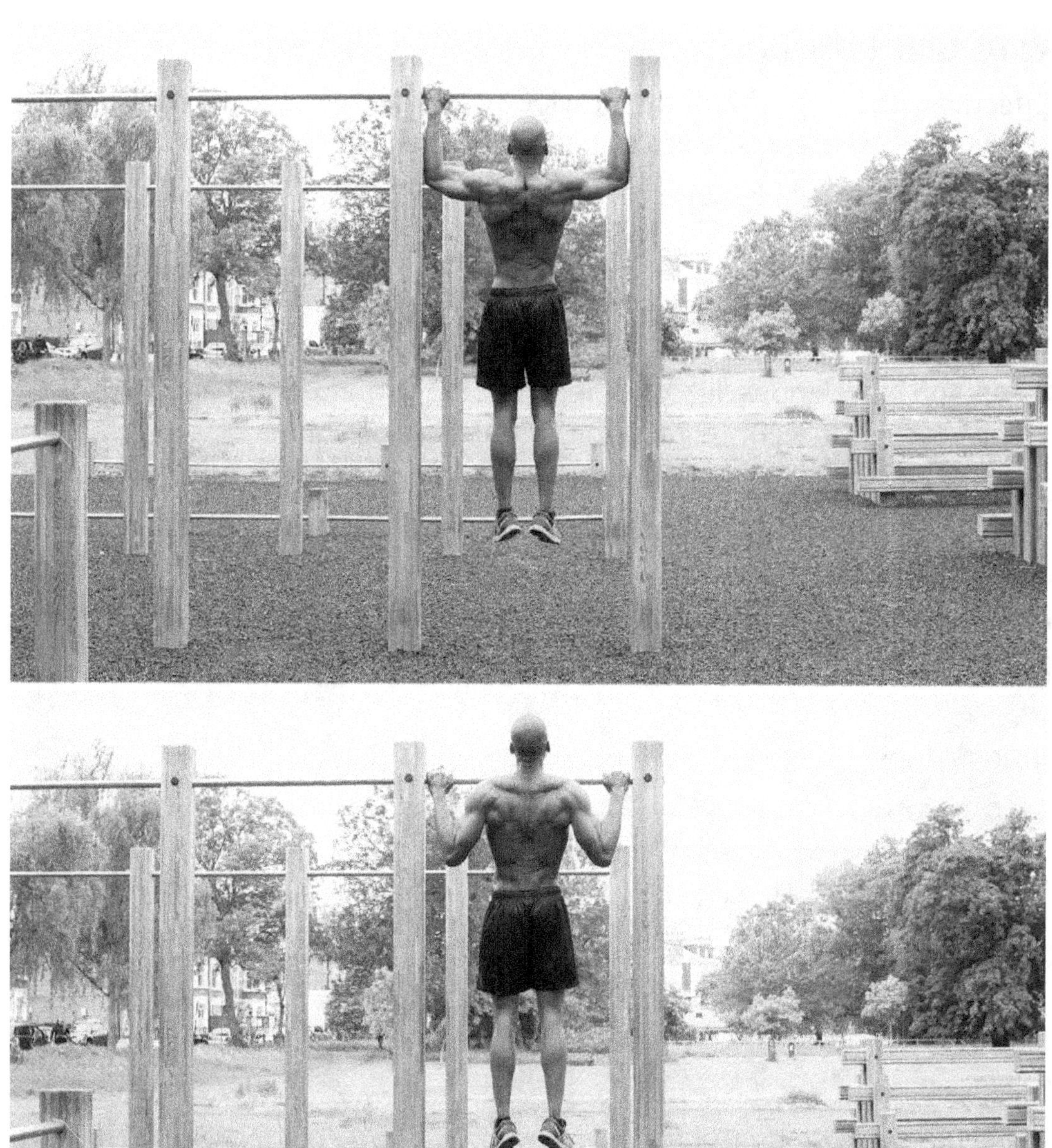

MUSCLE-UPS

When you are comfortable with all variations of the pushing and pulling exercises we've presented on the bar up to this point then you are ready to take on a truly versatile and astonishingly effective combination of both. Prepare for war, comrade, this one's tough!

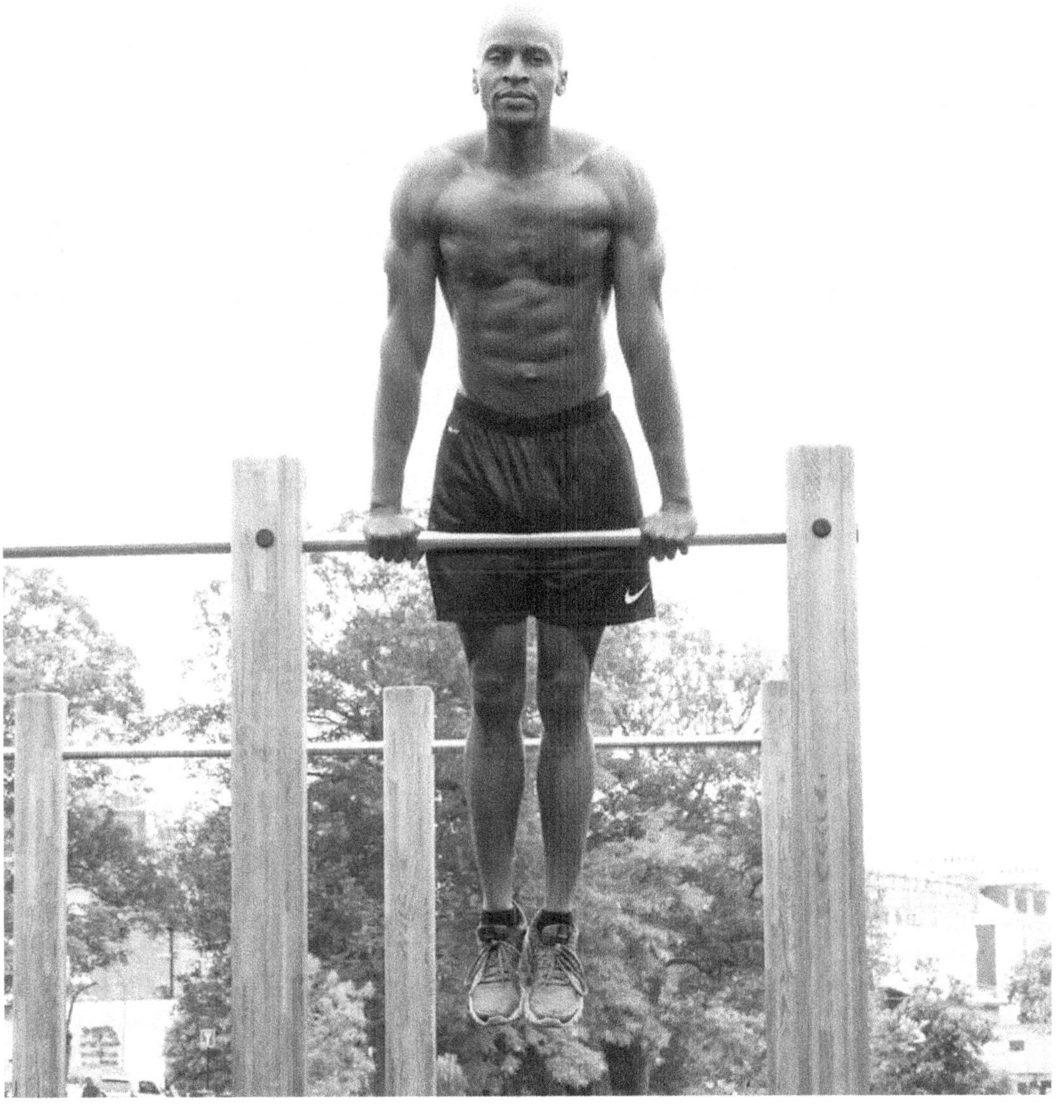

STANDARD MUSCLE-UP

There is nothing 'standard' about the amount of strength required to perform this one without swinging around like a safari park chimp. Work up to it and you will get there!

Perform: 3-4 sets of 6-10 reps.

You will need: a pull-up bar.

1. Grab that bar using an overhand grip, hands approximately shoulder width apart.

2. Perform a pull-up, hauling yourself up to the bar with as much power as possible.

3. In one movement, loosen your grip slightly, rotate your hands forward so you can prepare to push in the second step (see the false grip next for more).

4. Without stopping, push yourself up as high as possible, locking your elbows at the top of the movement.

5. Perform the process in reverse to lower yourself back down and complete 1 rep. Do not drop off the bar.

Variations:

• If you are struggling to generate enough power to bring your chin above the bar, you can use your feet for a little added momentum. At step 2, swing your feet forward very slightly, and then use the backwards momentum which follows to pull yourself up to the bar with as much power as possible.

• You can also practice each part individually and then piece them together over time to make it simpler.

This exercise will take a lot of practice – the aim is to complete the whole thing in one fluid motion without using momentum, so don't rely on that to get by.

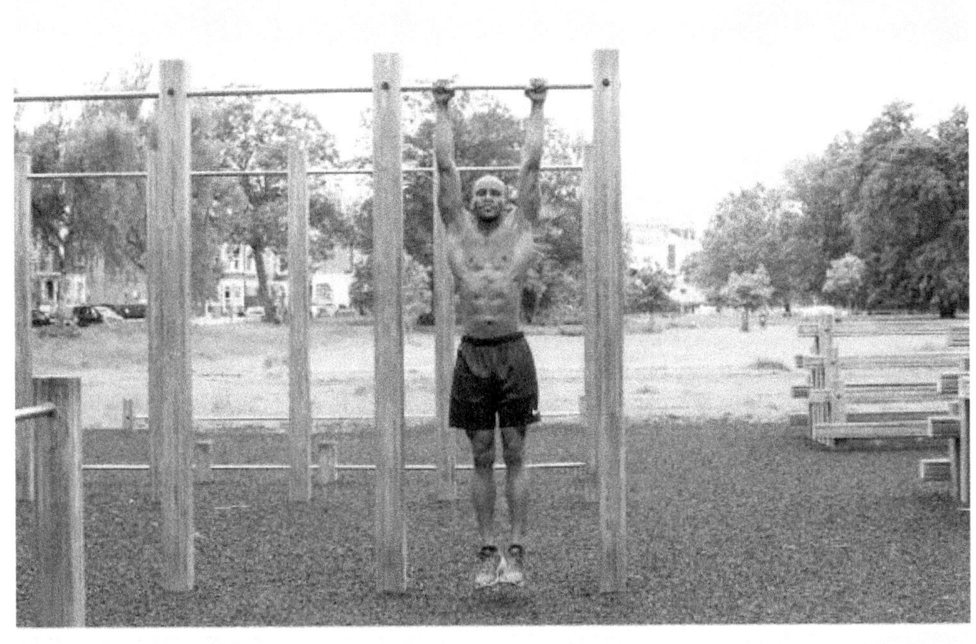

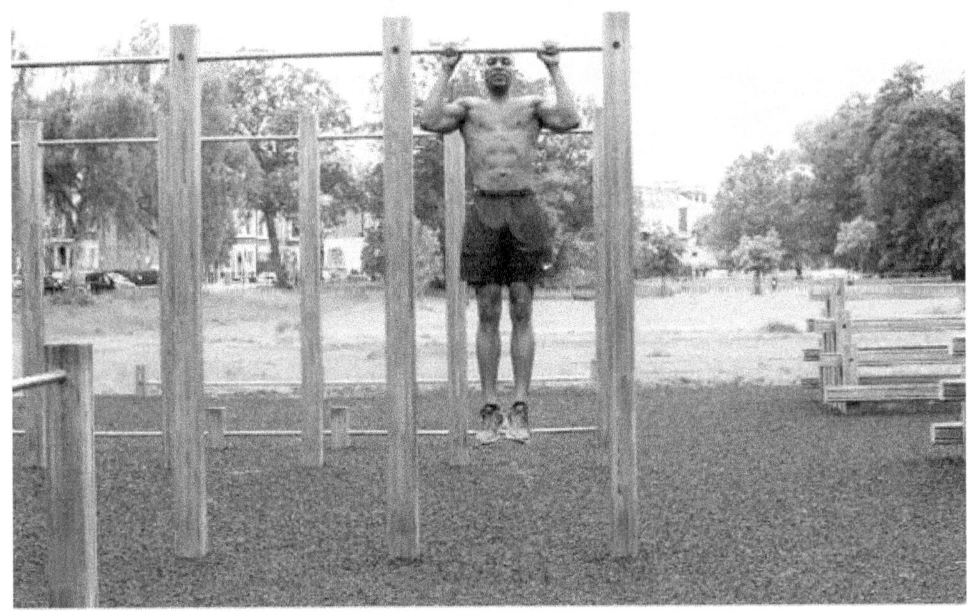

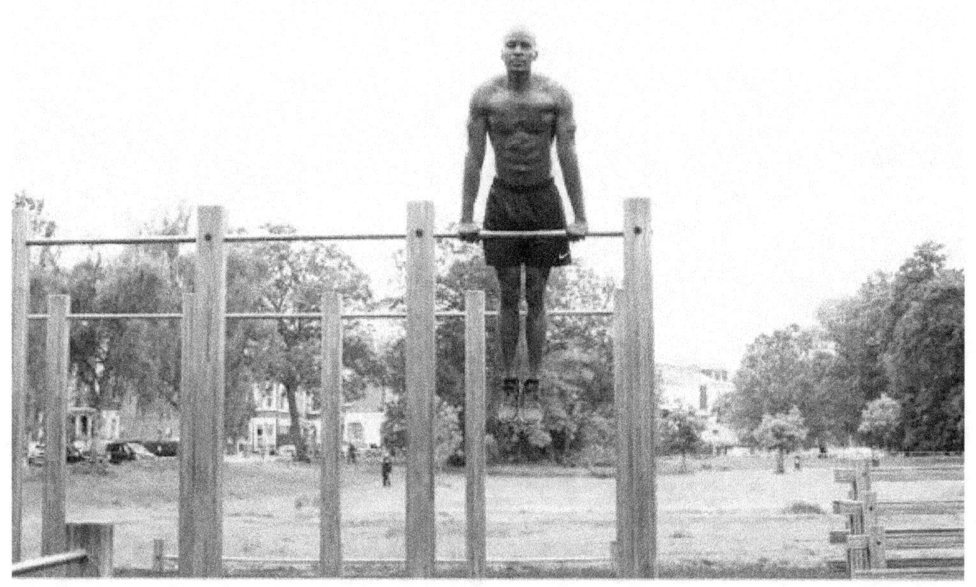

HANDSTANDS

Consider the strength your legs must possess to carry you around all day, and now think about how great it would be if you could transfer that level of strength to the upper body, too. This is exactly what we aim to achieve through handstand exercises. Let's go!

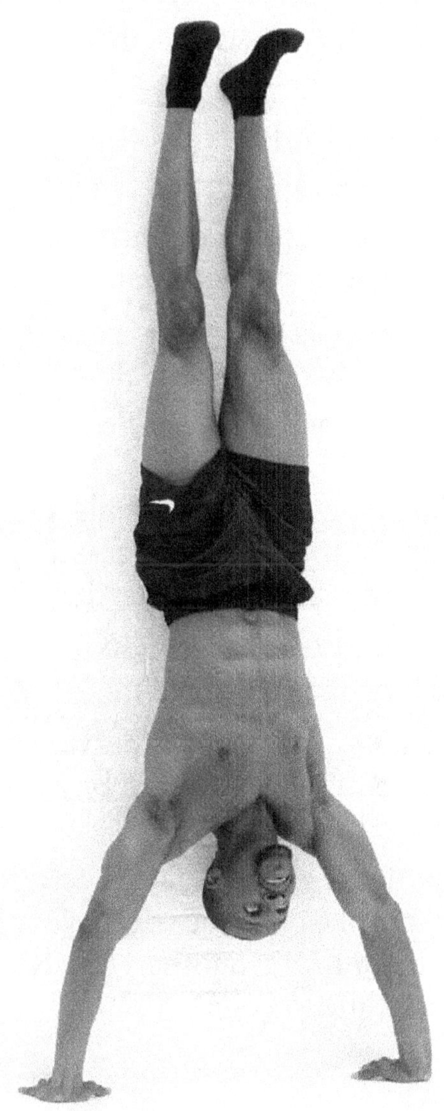

WALL WALKS

If you haven't performed a handstand recently or even at all then this is the perfect exercise to build up your strength at the same time as your confidence.

You should be somewhat familiar with this exercise from the wall push-ups presented previously. The difference here is that we'll be taking it up a little higher and transferring a greater load to the shoulders, arms and hands in prep for performing handstands.

Perform: maximum hold time possible.

You will need: a solid wall that can take your weight.

1. Get into a regular push-up position but instead of placing your feet on the floor, place them flat against the bottom of the wall.

2. Keeping your arms and legs as straight as possible and your core pulled in tight, begin to walk your feet up the wall in small steps. As they get higher you will also need to move your hands backwards to support your bodyweight.

3. When you have walked up as high as possible, aim to hold this position for a few seconds before slowly walking back down to the start, again aiming to keep your arms, legs and body straight.

As your strength and confidence increases you can walk higher and extend the amount of time you hold the top position.

Super important: This is a nice, gentle introduction to being upside-down, but can still be quite disorientating. Talk to a physician to ensure it is safe for you.

Take it slow, and at the first sign of dizziness or discomfort, come down and stay seated for a little while until you regain your composure. Don't try to stand up or jump straight into another exercise after being upside-down, as your body needs time to adjust.

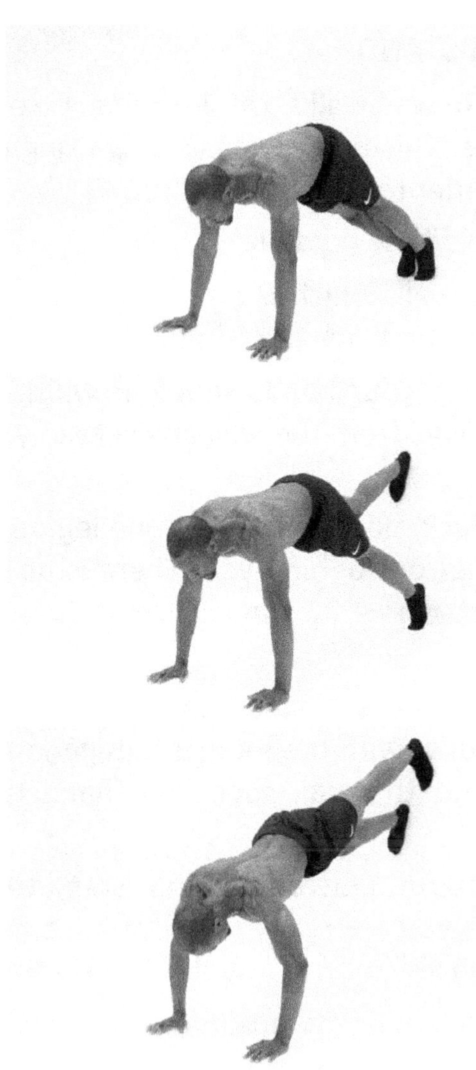

WALL SUPPORT HANDSTAND

Not to be confused with wall walks, this is the next step in the progression of handstand exercises. This time, instead of walking up the wall you will 'kick' up against it in order to get into position.

Perform: maximum hold time possible.

You will need: a solid wall, which can take your weight and a spotter if you're new to this (just don't kick them in the face!)

1. Facing the wall, place your hands shoulder width apart on the floor, approximately a foot away from the wall and spread your fingers out wide for balance.

2. Get into 'starting block' pose by tucking one leg up close to your chest and extending the other out behind you. There is no right or wrong foot here, simply find what works for you or switch it up as and when you please.

3. Use the leg that is tucked underneath you to kick upwards while swinging the back leg over with the momentum generated. This should be enough to get you into the wall supported handstand position if you commit to it.

If you are nervous about performing this step, try kicking up small amounts at first. When you are ready to go for it, commit with confidence that the wall WILL catch you, or use a spotter if necessary.

4. When you are in the handstand position, hold it for as long as possible, keeping your whole body locked straight. Stay calm and breathe normally.

5. To descend, keep your arms locked and drop one leg followed by the other. Try to control this movement rather than simply dropping down like a sack of spuds as this will build even greater strength.

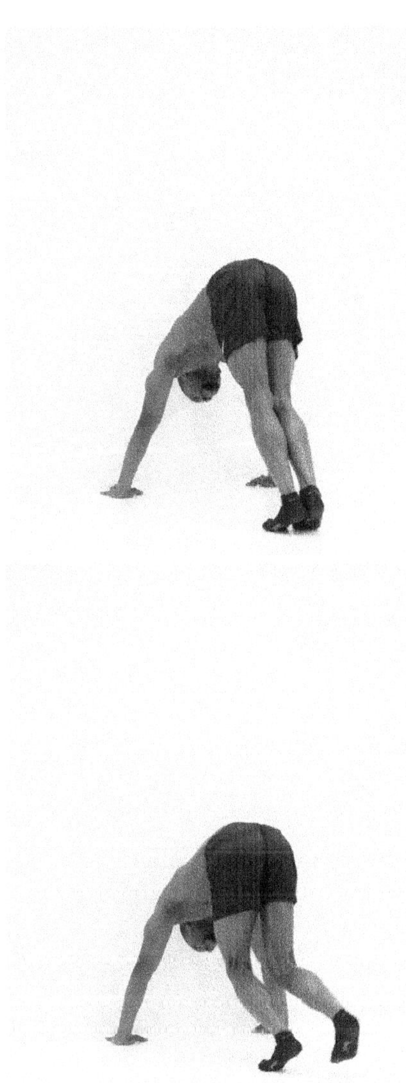

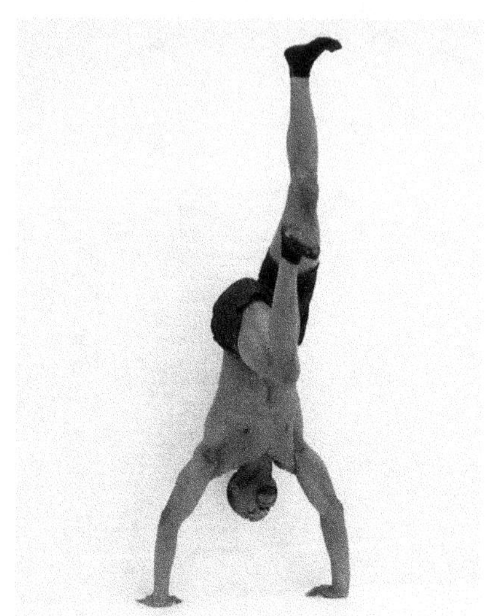

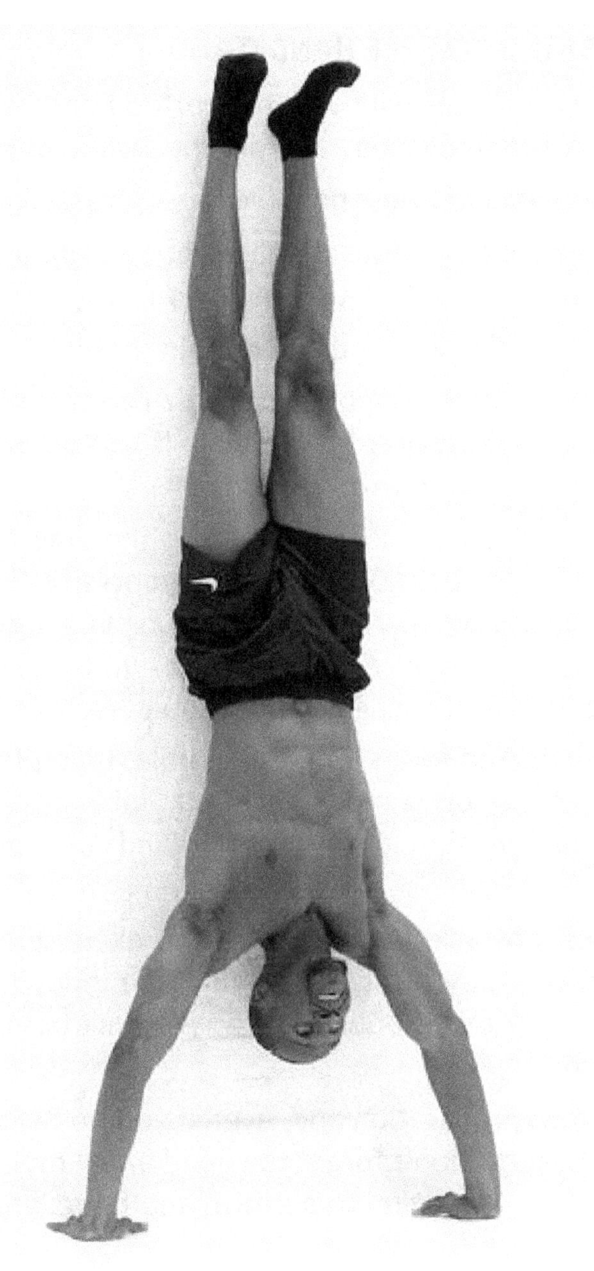

WALL HANDSTAND TO FREE HANDSTAND

Once you're comfortable with wall-supported handstands, it's time to begin the process of moving away from the wall to develop your balance.

Perform: maximum hold time possible.

You will need: a solid wall that can take your weight and a spotter if you're new to this (again try not to hit them on your way up!)

1. Kick up into a wall handstand and remain there.

2. With as much force as possible, push down with your fingertips to encourage your feet away from the wall. If this doesn't work, push away from the wall VERY softly with your feet.

3. When your feet are no longer touching the wall try to balance in this position for as long as possible. If you find yourself falling back towards the wall, or overbalancing, correct this by pushing down hard with your fingertips. If you experience the opposite, under-balancing, try bending your elbows a little and engaging your shoulders to assist.

4. Hold the handstand for as long as possible. If you fall back into the wall or down to the floor, simply get back into position and try again. Remember, your feet should stay together and come away from the wall as shown.

NB: The biggest obstacle to performing this exercise can often be mental. Fear of failure or injury often causes us to be indecisive, but you needn't be concerned with this if you are in a safe environment and / or have a spotter with you.

Trust in your own preparation and, even if you do fall back down, it will be a controlled descent. Don't forget to spend a few moments regaining your composure before getting up to perform another exercise!

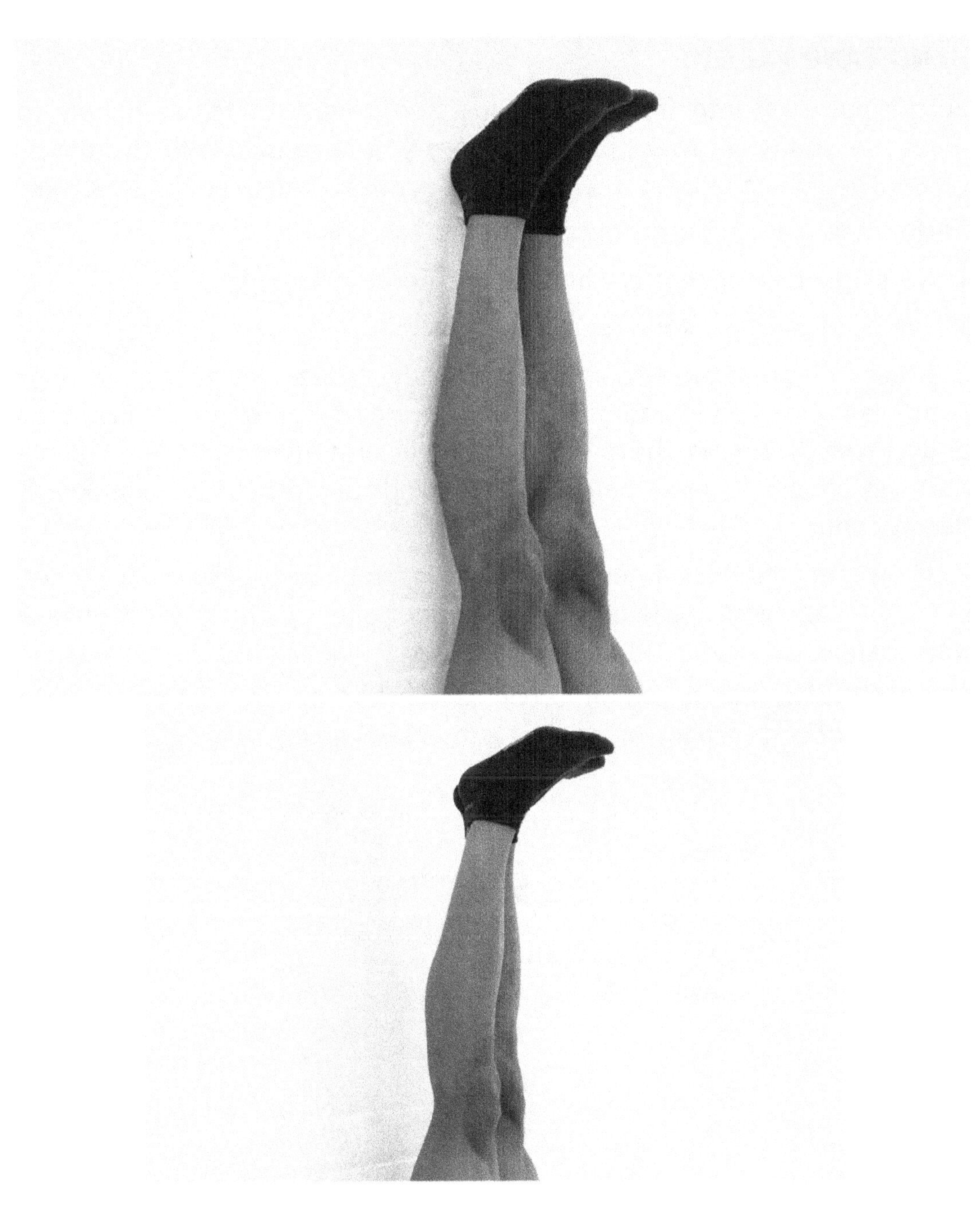

HANDSTAND BAILOUT

Before you dive into free handstands it is important to learn how to recover if you begin to topple over. Once you have mastered this move, you will be able to take on free handstands without the need for a spotter.

Perform: as many repetitions as needed to feel confident.

You will need: an open space and matted flooring if possible.

1. Kick up into a handstand (or attempt to!)

2. When you go into overbalance – that is your legs and feet going over your head – take one hand off the floor. By doing this you will cause your body to pivot around the hand that is still rooted to the floor. People normally choose to keep their strongest hand rooted but find what works best for you.

3. Allow the momentum generated to bring your body around, and then place the hand you lifted up back to the floor and let your legs come back down safely.

Practice this technique until it becomes a reflex and you will never again have to suffer the pain or embarrassment of going down like a Jenga tower!

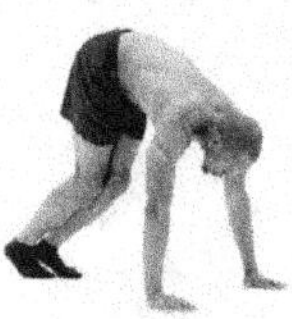

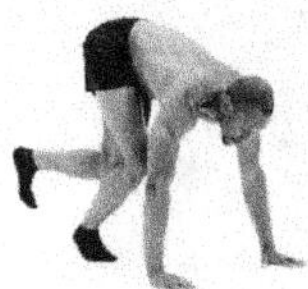

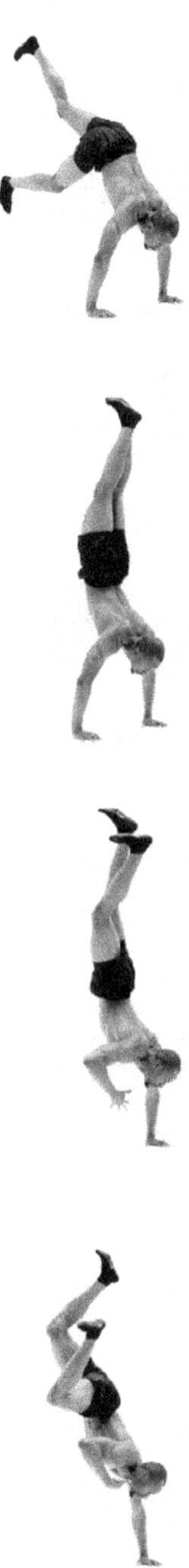

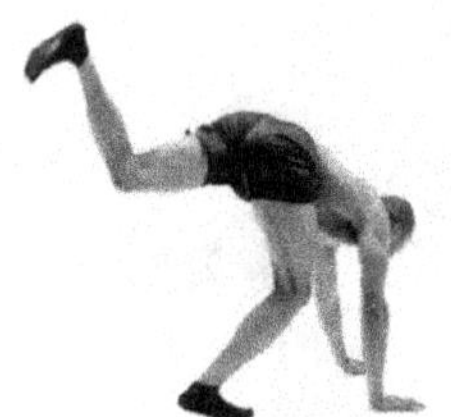

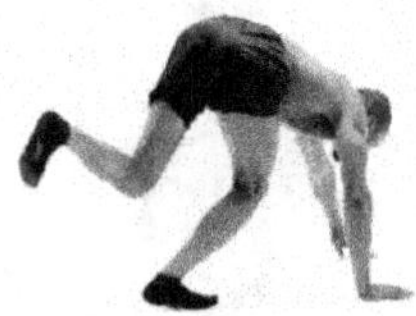

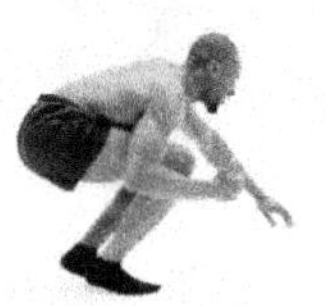

FLOOR / FREE HANDSTAND

The final stage of the standard handstand is the free handstand. Don't worry if this seems daunting at first – you have your escape strategy so you'll be able to bail out if things don't go to plan right away.

Perform: maximum hold time possible.

You will need: a clear space and matted flooring if possible.

1. Ensuring there is plenty of room around you, kick up into a handstand.

2. Your feet will likely travel over and past your head causing you to overbalance. You can correct this in the same way as before, by pushing down hard with your fingertips.

3. Hold the handstand for as long as possible and then perform a controlled descent.

As one of the hardest movements this is really venturing into advanced calisthenics so don't be disheartened if it takes a while to learn.

Depending on your level of ability it may take a matter of weeks, months or even up to a year or more to truly perfect the handstand.

The great thing about calisthenics is that you will still be building incredible strength while you learn with the simpler movements shown before.

You will reach your goals much quicker by accepting where you are and taking a step back than trying to rush ahead with poor form.

Up next we're going to continue progressing towards intermediate upper body work with some of the essential levers. !

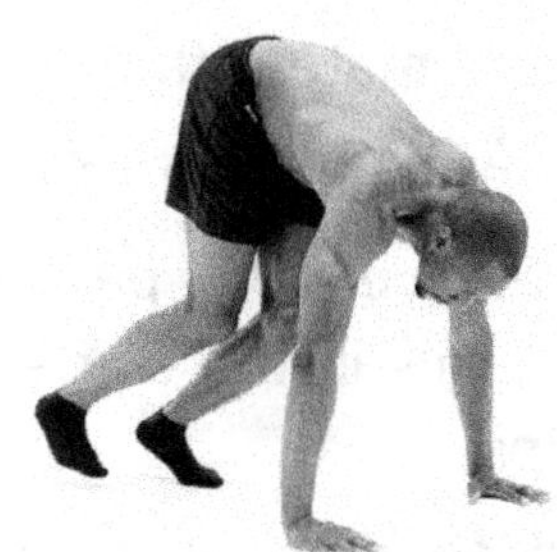

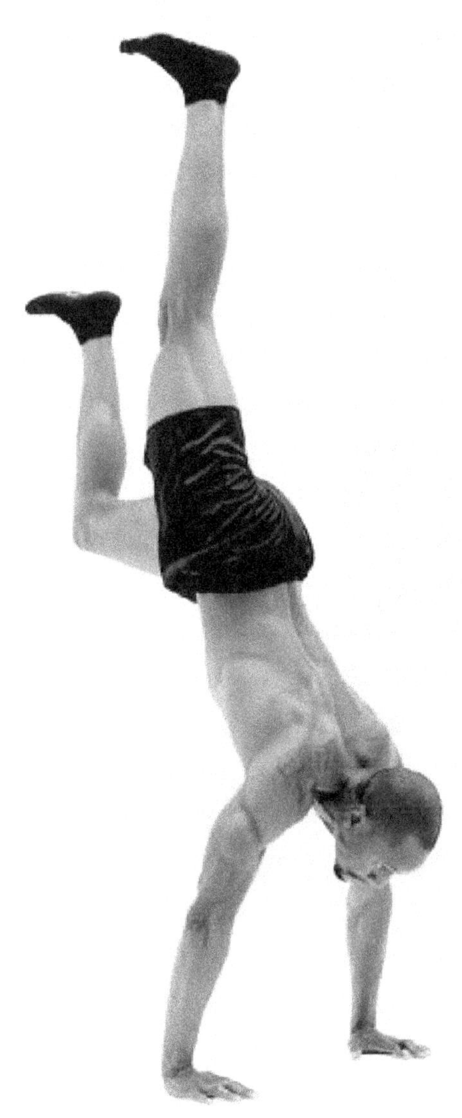

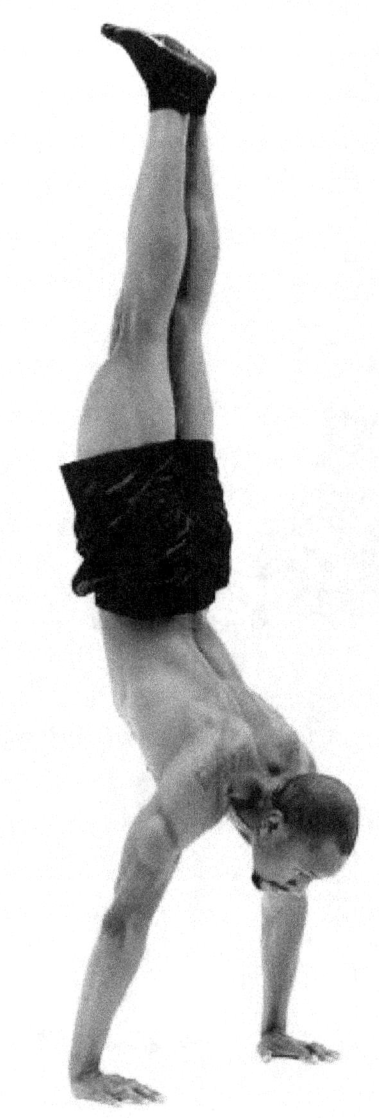

UPPER BODY LEVERS

After all you've been through you would be forgiven for thinking you have 'completed' calisthenics. However, we're just getting started! So far we've largely been in motion, and it's now time to delve into isometric - or static - exercises. This is where calisthenics comes into its own. Prepare to level up, comrade. The road to SUPERHUMAN continues!

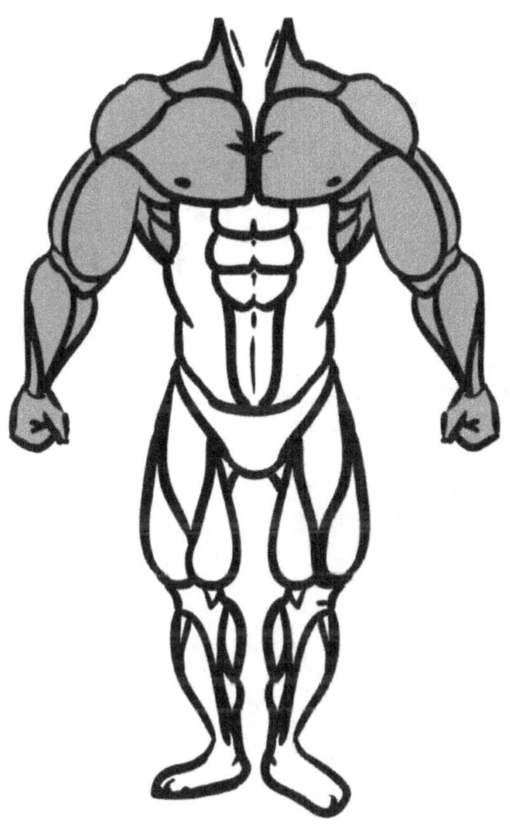

LEVERS

Levers take us into intermediate territory, so we won't be aiming for the more advanced exercises here. Instead we will build a solid foundation based on the key elements you will need to build upon later. Repetition is key here. Keep holding position for as long as you can and with time and patience you will achieve mastery.

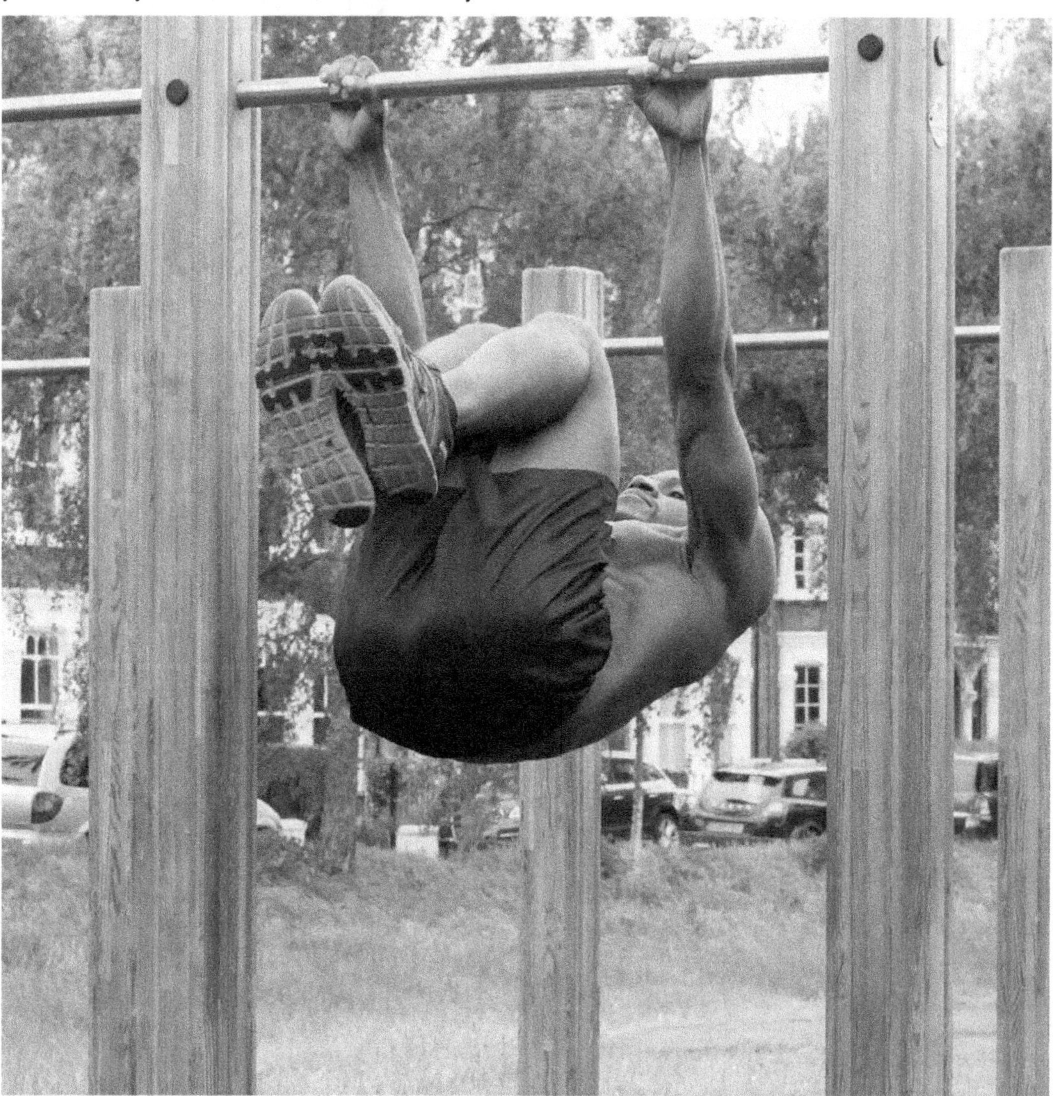

STRAIGHT PULL

As we branch into the field of the front lever, it's important to develop the concept of pulling down on the bar without bending at the elbows. To practice this skill, work on this straightforward vertical pull maneuver.

Perform: 10-20 second hold time.

You will need: pull-up bar.

1. Assume the standard pull-up position by grasping the bar with an overhand grip and keeping your hands shoulder width apart.

2. Begin from a dead hang, with arms completely locked out. Now pull your shoulders away and down from your ears. Remember to keep your arms straight!

3. Now begin to lean back a little while pulling hard on the bar. Try to close the angle between your arms and chest. As you get stronger, the gap will close further and further until you are able to get closer to the full front lever.

4. Hold for as long as possible, then drop off the bar and reset.

NB: If you are going into this exercise without any prior practice on the bar, then you will likely find it impossible.

We've mentioned several times that this is a progressive calisthenics guide, so if you cannot complete this movement please go back and cover the previous exercises.

As with all foundation exercises, straight pulls will take great patience to conquer. Once you have achieved perfect form, though, you will find the following exercises come much more naturally to you.

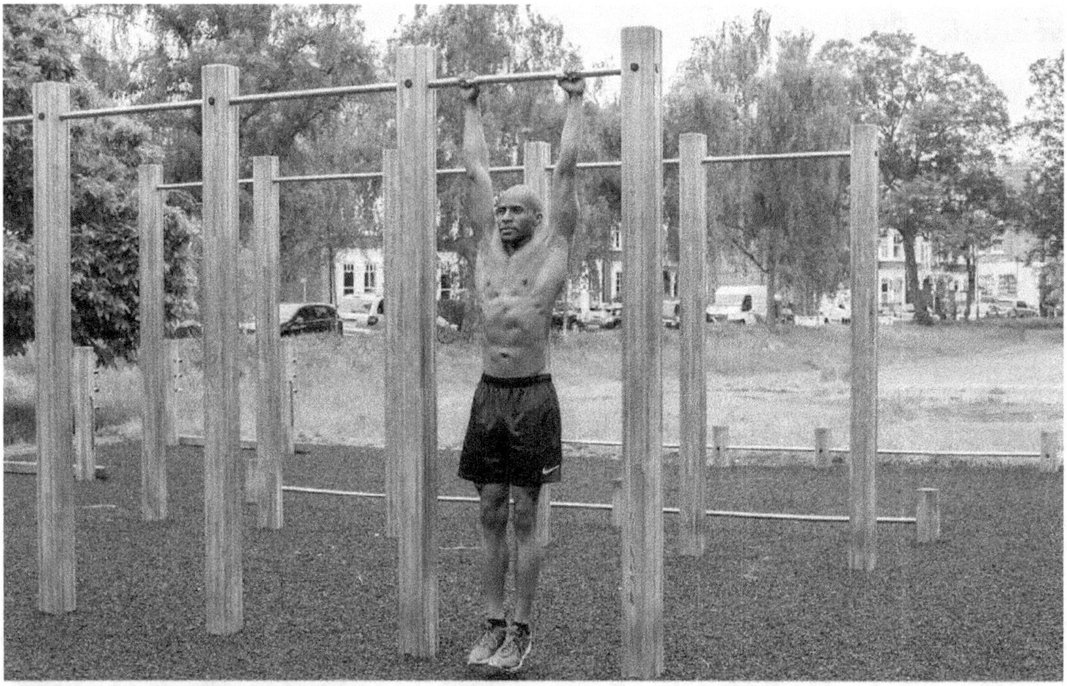

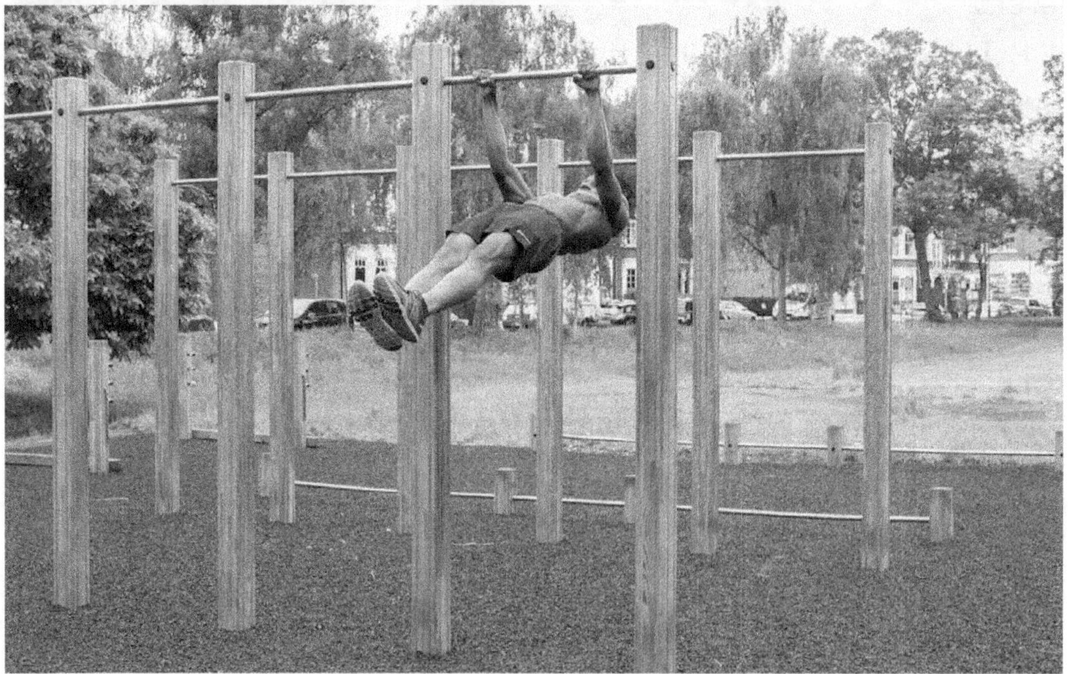

TUCK FRONT LEVER

When you've nailed the straight pull, it's time to tackle the front tuck front lever. We'll begin to engage the core with this position, keeping your legs close and tucked up to your chest to limit the strain to begin with. This will later serve as a solid foundation for the full front lever.

Perform: 10-20 second hold time.

You will need: pull-up bar.

1. Assume the standard pull-up position, and allow yourself to hang with your arms completely locked out.

2. Engage your core, and pull your knees up to your chest. You should pivot so that your back is facing the ground.

3. Continue to pull down on the bar with your arms locked out, and hold for as long as possible. When you feel strong enough to up your game, let your knees come away from your chest so your hips align with your shoulders, achieving a straight back.

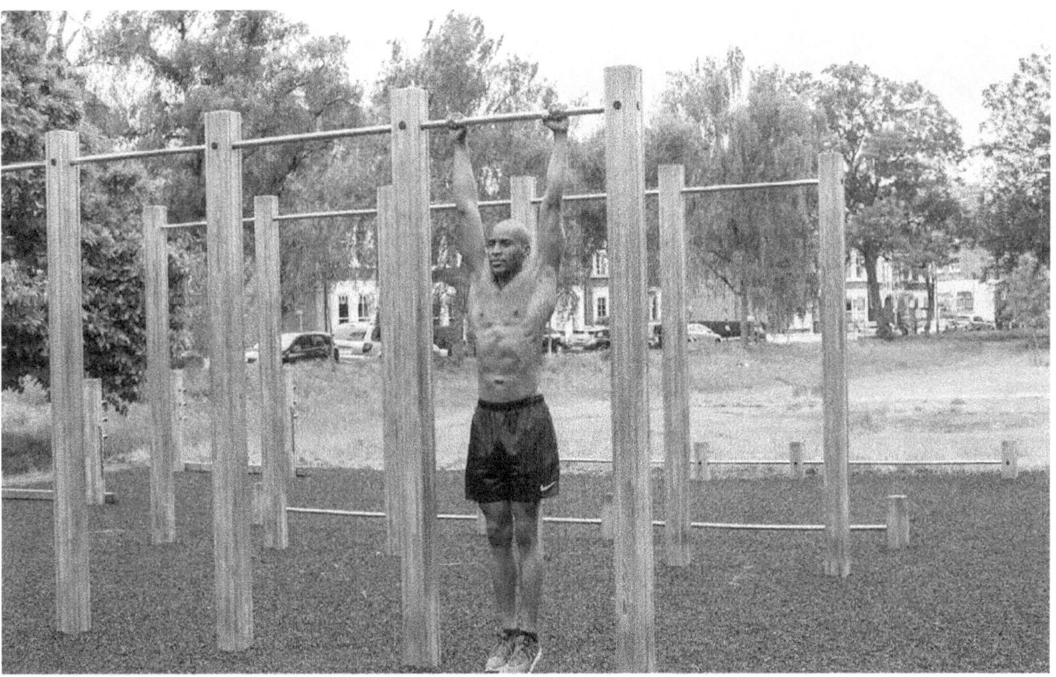

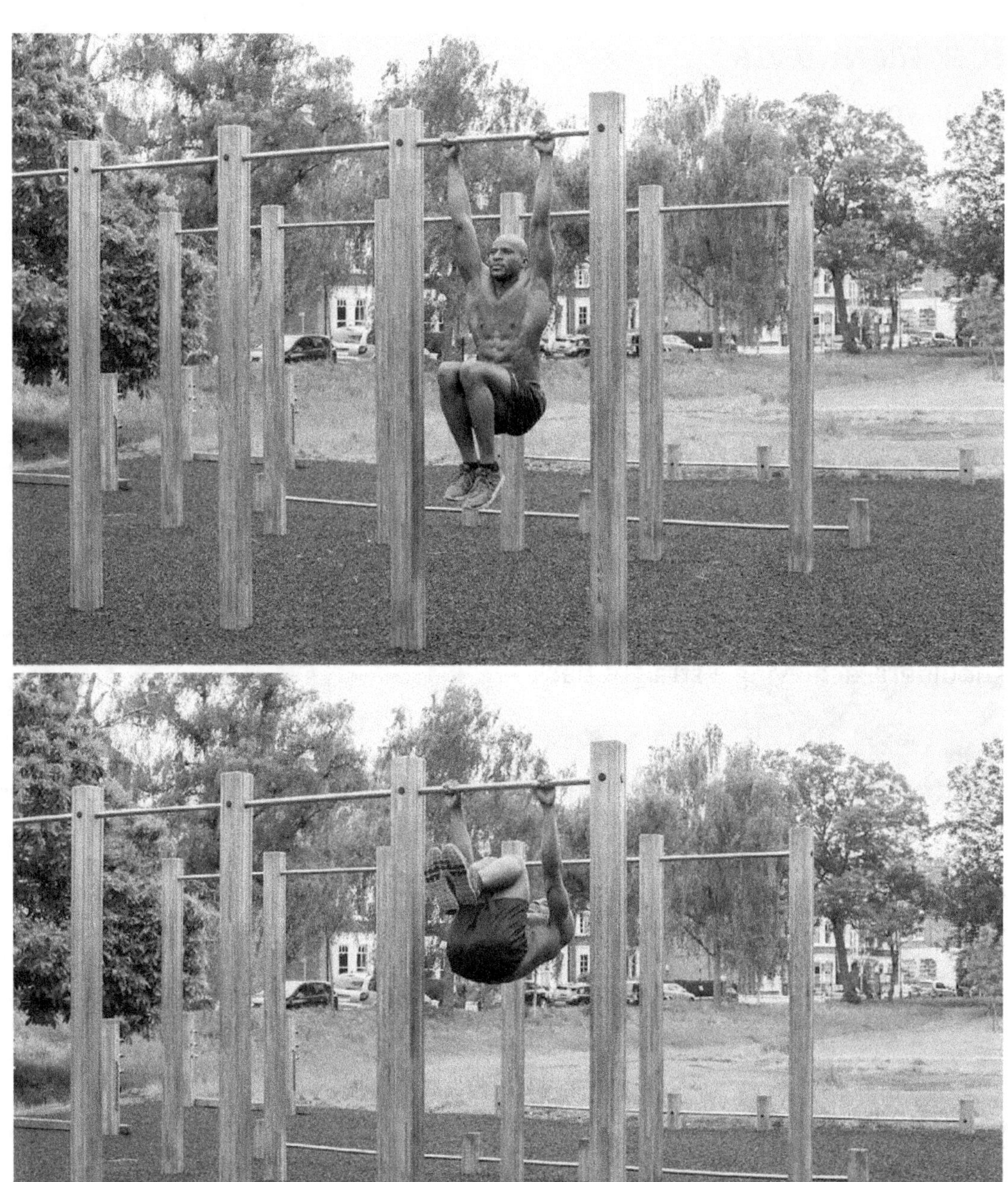

SKIN THE CAT

Before you can begin to learn back levers you'll first need to focus on your shoulder mobility and strength. This position will feel uncomfortable and unstable to start with, so take it slow and concentrate on increasing your range of motion.

Perform: 10-15 second hold time.

You will need: pull-up bar.

1. Grasp the bar in the standard pull-up position with locked out arms and an overhand grip.

2. Now engage your core and bring your legs up in a leg raise, while at the same time leaning backwards.

3. Bend your knees enough to bring your legs all the way through the gap between your arms, continuing your backward momentum.

4. Carry on rotating until you are facing forwards once more, with your legs hanging underneath you, and hold for as long as possible

Remember: This book is designed to teach calisthenics in a progressive manner. If you're finding something too difficult, don't try to 'power through.'

If you are truly committed to calisthenics then you must understand that it is a gradual learning curve. Take a step back, assess your progress and, if necessary, revisit earlier exercises to work on your foundational strength.

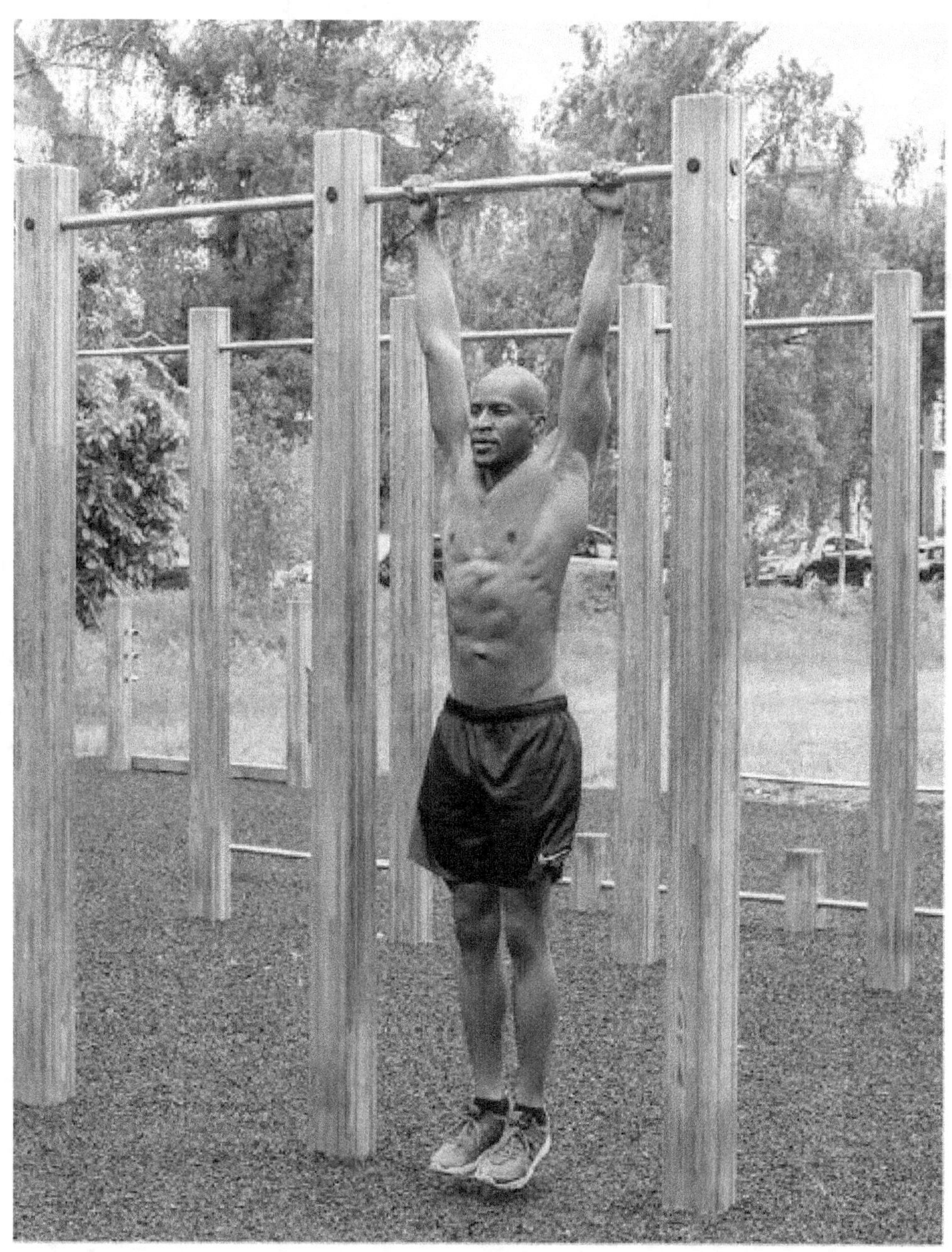

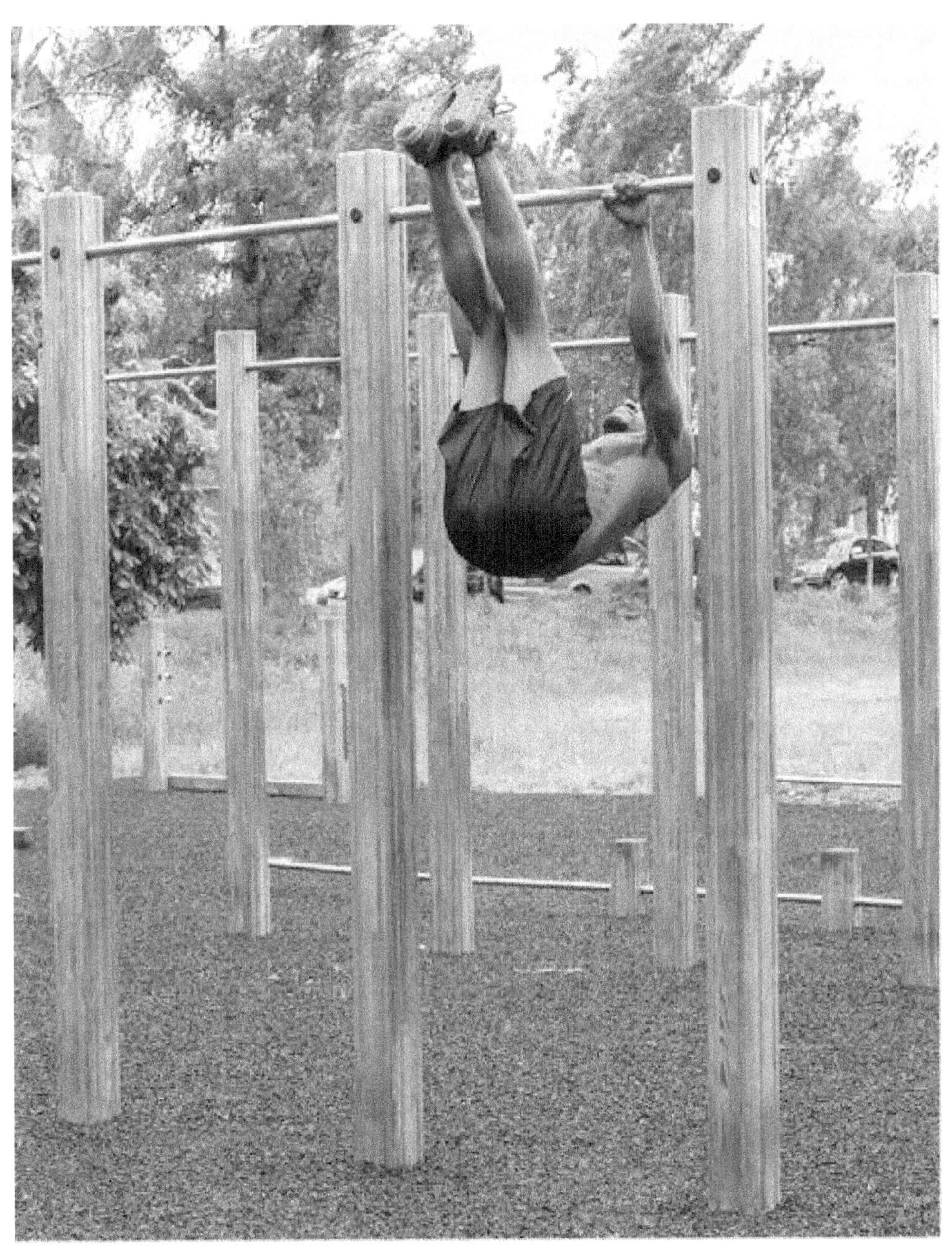

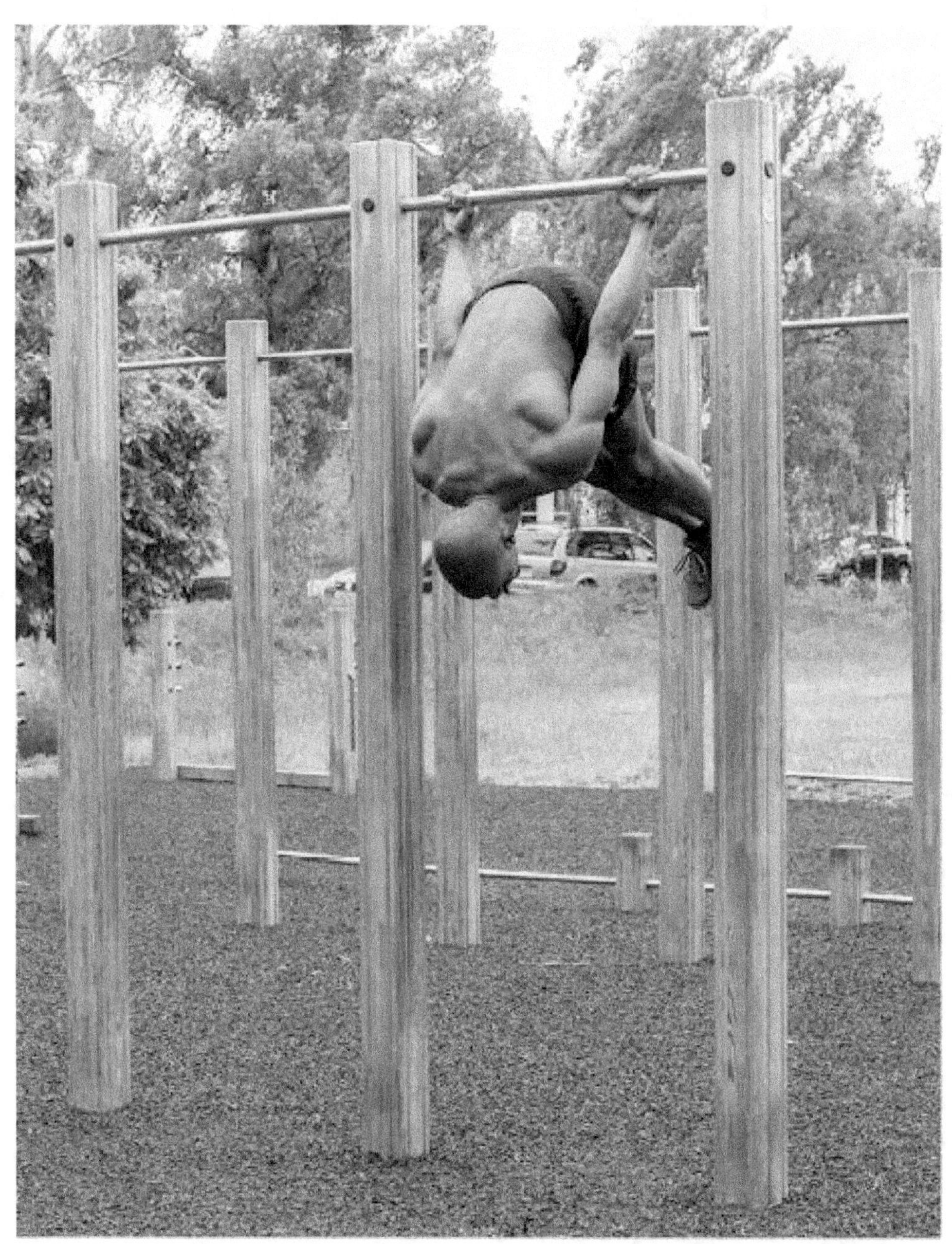

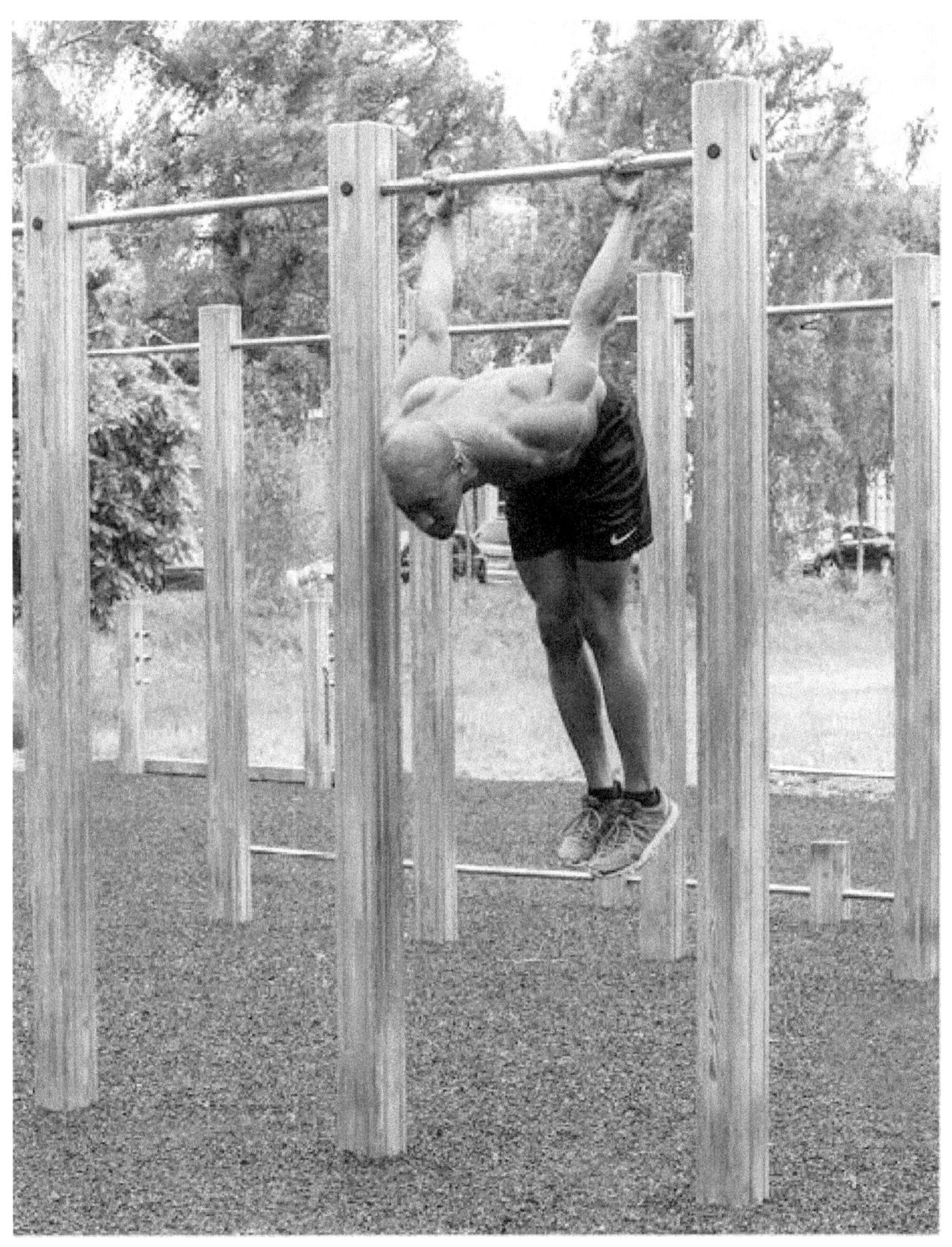

TUCK HALF LEVER

This exercise will familiarize you with parallettes and provide a basis for learning the full half lever and other upper body and core moves. You will need to nail this before you can move on to more difficult positions such as the ones in our more advanced books.

Perform: 20-30 second hold time.

You will need: parallettes or two other sturdy, raised platforms.

1. Position yourself between the parallettes, grasp them, and push yourself up. Your hands and elbows should be directly under your shoulders and in line with your hips.

2. Now engage your core and keep your knees bent at 90 degrees. Lift your legs until your thighs are at 90 degrees to your torso, or horizontal.

3. Hold for long as possible.

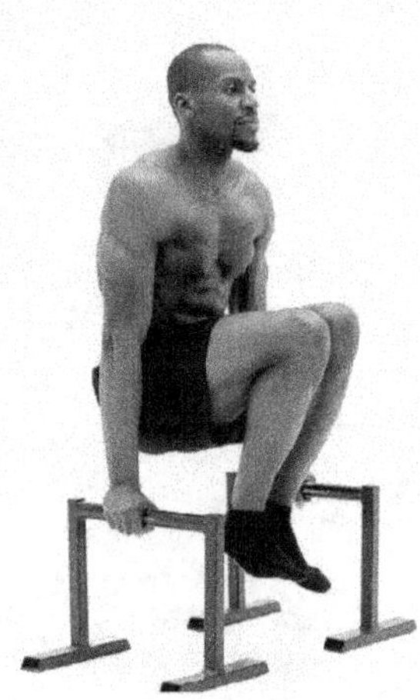

PLANCHE LEAN

This simple pose is your starting point for building the upper body strength and stability required to pull off the various other planche moves covered later down the line.

Perform: 3-4 sets of 10-20 second holds.

1. Get into regular push-up position with your elbows locked.

2. Slowly walk your feet forward, keeping your hands rooted, so that your shoulders move past and in front of your hands.

3. Stretch out your scapulae as if you were trying to get your shoulders to touch in front of you and raise your spine as high as possible.

4. Once you are at maximum stretch, hold to complete one set.

Variation: Use parallettes instead of the floor.

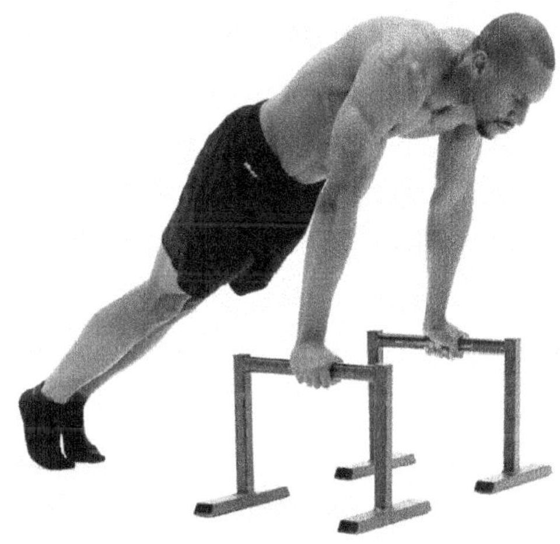

FROG STAND

The next progression in the lever exercise group is the frog stand, which helps condition your hands, wrists and arms and upper body in preparation for further progress.

Perform: 10-20 second hold time.

1. Place your hands flat on the floor in front of you, fingers facing forward in the most natural position for you.

2. Crouching down like a frog, bring your knees forward and rest them against the outsides of your elbows.

3. Push down hard with your hands and slowly let your feet lift off the floor, leaning forward slightly if it helps your balance.

4. Hold this position until you reach the allotted time. If you can't complete the allotted time, perform as many sets as it takes to do e.g. 2 x 10 seconds.

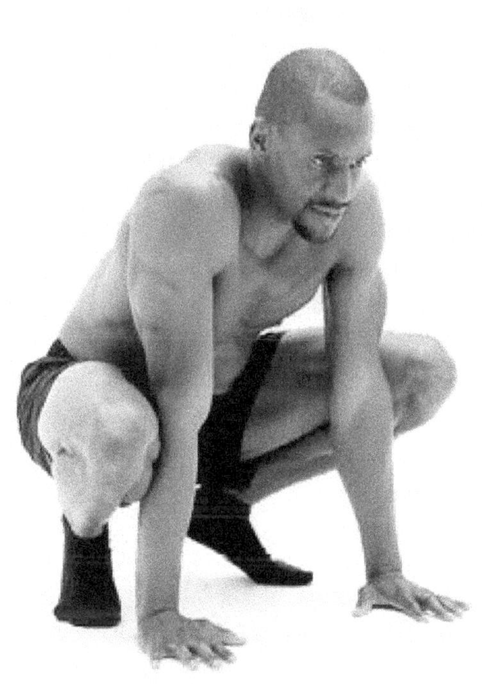

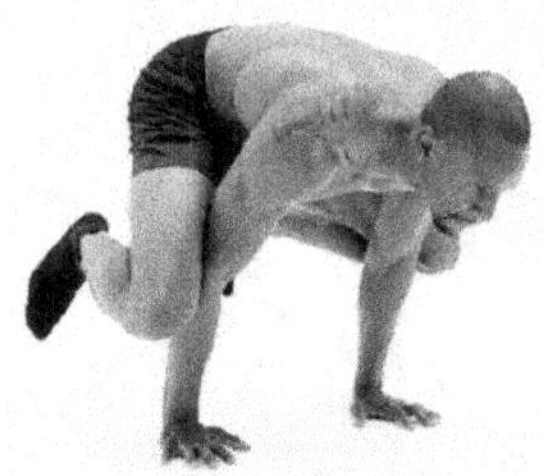

TUCK PLANCHE

We are well into intermediate territory here, so be sure to nail what has come before!

Perform: 10-20 second hold time.

You will need: parallettes if you wish.

1. Place your hands on the parallettes and lift your feet off the ground.

2. Bring your knees up towards your chest, supporting your bodyweight on your wrists.

3. Lean forward until your upper bodyweight counterbalances your lower bodyweight and try to hold this position. Once again, perform as many sets as it takes to hit your allotted time.

Variations:

• Ditch the parallettes and go on the floor!

• You can also perform the exercise with your fingers pointing backwards to engage your biceps more if doing this on the floor.

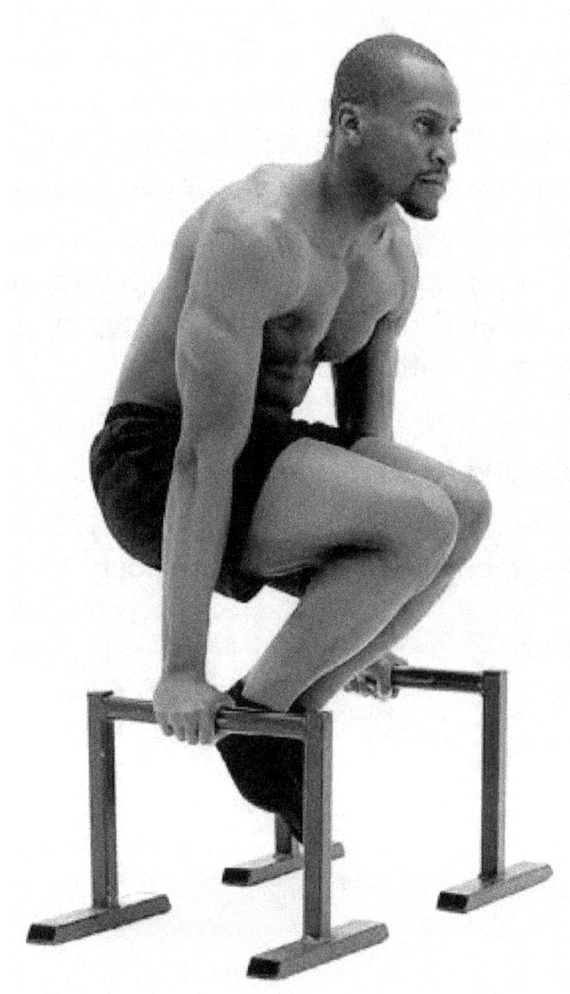

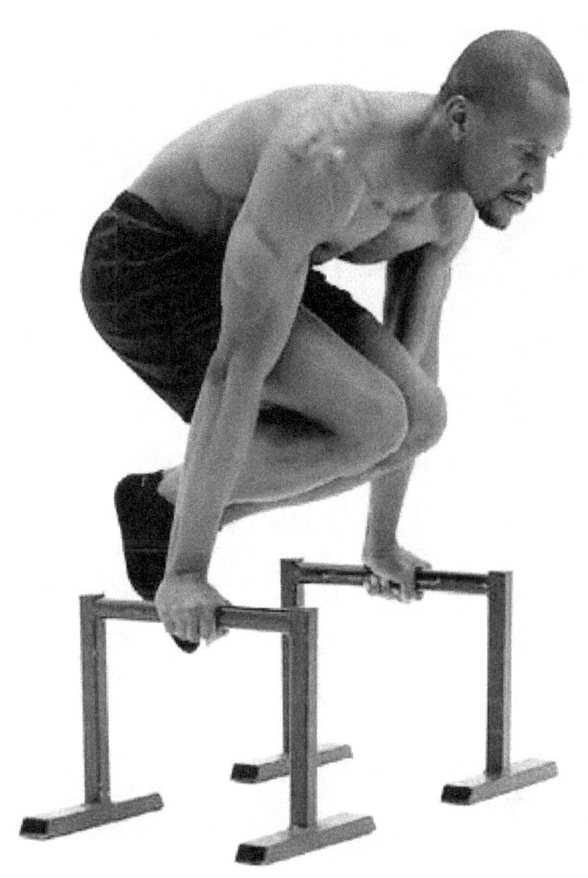

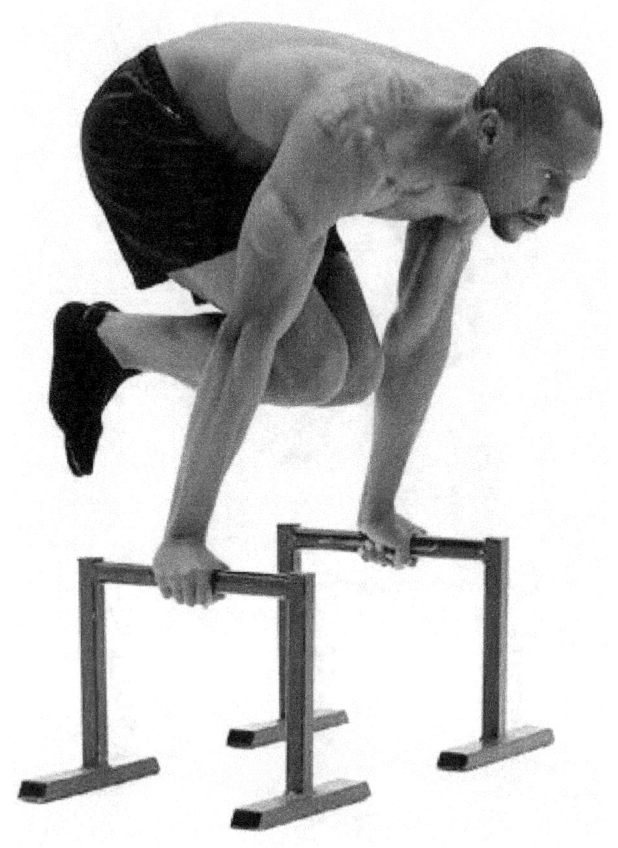

STRAIGHT BACK PLANCHE

When you can hold the tuck planche for approximately 30 seconds, you can graduate to the flat back variation. The subtle but crucial difference being that we will now maintain a completely flat back during the hold, which will engage your core and shoulders.

Perform: 10-20 second hold time.

1. Place your hands on the ground approx shoulder width apart, and raise yourself into the tuck planche position.

2. Once there, continue to raise your hips until they are at about the same level as your shoulders, so your back should be straight.

3. Engage your core and lock out your arms, and maintain for allotted time.

The switch from curved to completely flat back may seem simple at face value, but it can be maddeningly difficult to master.

As a beginner working up to intermediate stage, remember to cut yourself some slack and appreciate how far you have already come.

This exercise falls under intermediate level, and once mastered you will be heading towards advanced. It is therefore reasonable to expect this to take a while to get right.

Calisthenics is all about patience so please do not be tempted to rush ahead. There is infinitely more value in getting the simple things down first.

That concludes our rundown of upper body exercises, so go ahead and celebrate a big win! Up next we'll get started on your core with some key exercises.

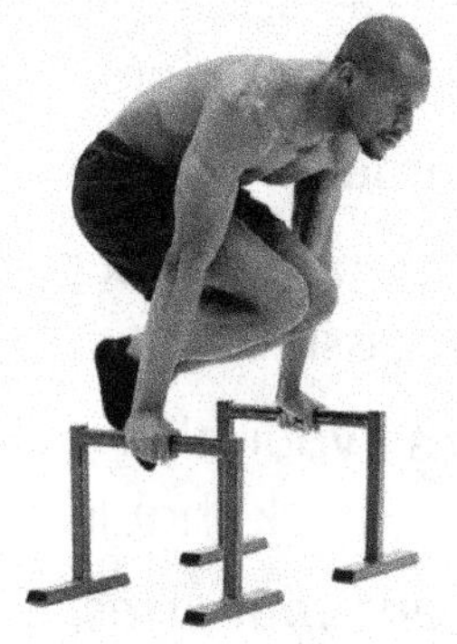

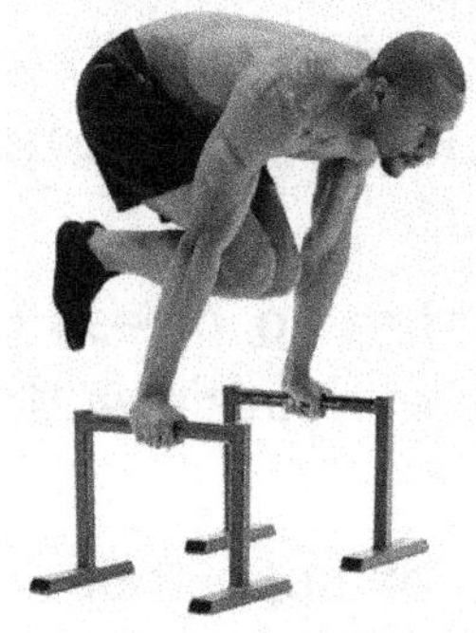

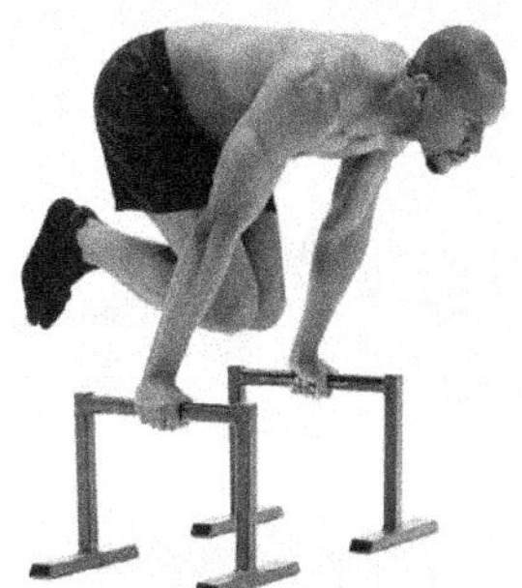

CORE

When it comes to calisthenics your core really is the star of the show. It may look like your upper and lower body are bearing the brunt of it, but everything is linked in the center so it is absolutely essential to pay special attention to developing core strength.

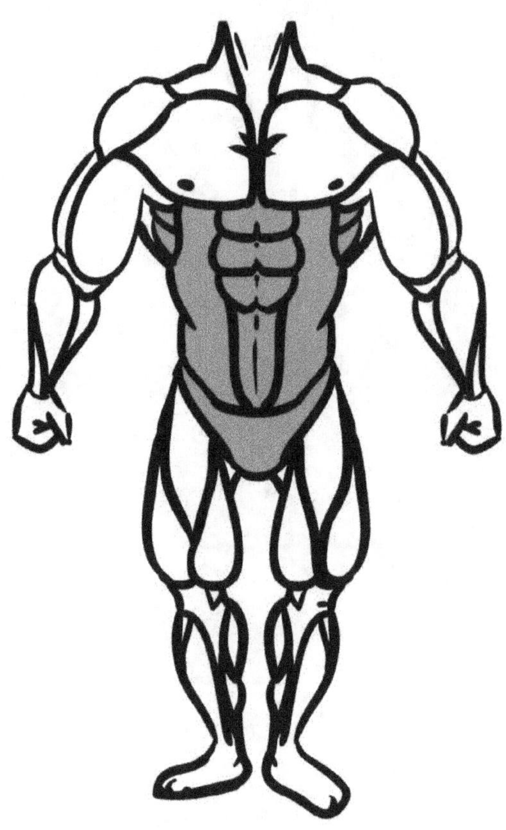

FUNDAMENTALS

Don't ignore the core! As the name suggests, your core is at the hub of all exercises, and you must keep it finely tuned if you want to build the perfect body. Progress through these fundamentals to achieve a popping six-pack and shredded stomach in quick time!

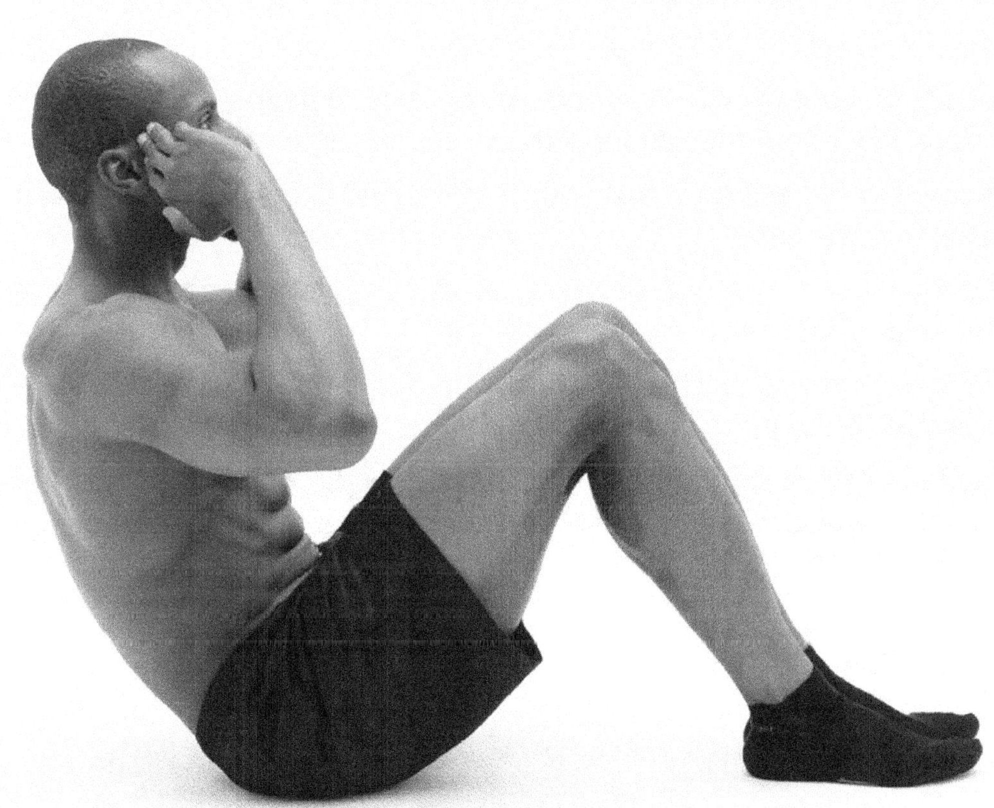

SIT-UP

This classic core exercise has been the foundation of training programs for as long as they have existed, so it's well worth mastering early on.

NB: Proper form is essential with all exercises, but it is especially important where the core is concerned, since you will also be calling your spine into action.

To maximize your results and avoid injury, always do as much as you can with the correct form instead of cheating to knock out another rep or two.

Perform: 3-4 sets of 10-20 reps.

1. Lie flat on your back with your knees bent at 90 degrees and feet flat on the floor. Place your toes under a secure surface if just starting out.

2. Place your fingertips against your temples and allow your arms to come parallel to the ground.

3. Contract your core and sit up as far as possible, aiming to bring your elbows past your knees.

4. When you have reached forward as far as possible, reverse the movement to complete one rep.

Variation: Have a buddy press your feet into the ground, or tuck them under something sturdy in order to generate greater leverage when you are just starting out.

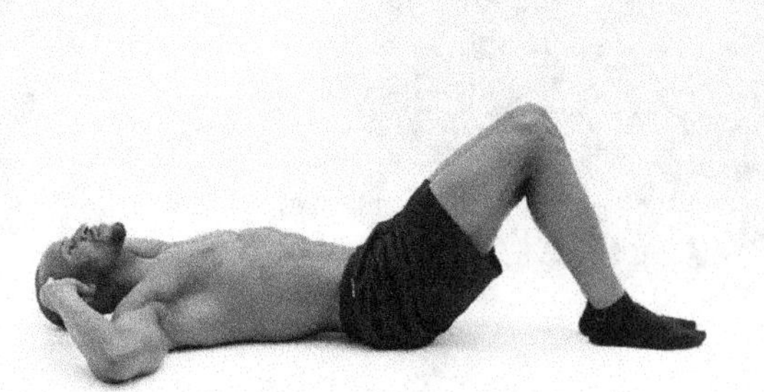

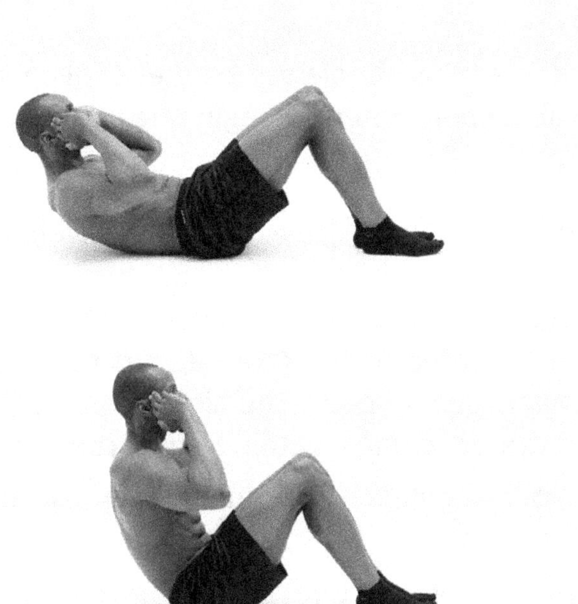

CRUNCH

The crunch is a fairly simple yet very effective way of strengthening your core and can be performed by beginners and experts alike.

Perform: 3-4 sets of 10-20 reps.

1. Lie on your back with your knees bent at approximately 90 degrees and your feet placed flat on the floor.

2. Place your hands loosely at the sides your head and, keeping your lower back and feet rooted to the ground, curl your shoulders and upper back forward towards your knees. The aim here is not to move far, but to feel a very concentrated 'crunch' within a small range of movement.

3. Lower your shoulders and upper back towards the ground again to complete one rep.

If you struggle to keep your feet flat on the ground during this exercise then place them under something secure until you are able to do the exercise properly.

Super important: do not use your hands to pull yourself up, as this will strain your neck. Instead, keep your chin tucked, hands loose and concentrate all the effort in your core.

If your neck is getting tired, it's because you are straining it to compensate for a weak core. Instead of yanking on your head, just perform fewer reps with the proper form.

Over time you will develop the core strength required to perform the allocated sets and reps, and you will find that your neck no longer seems to be a source of pain!

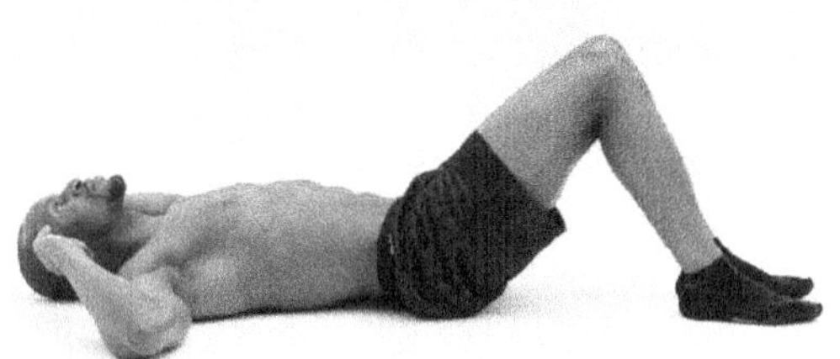

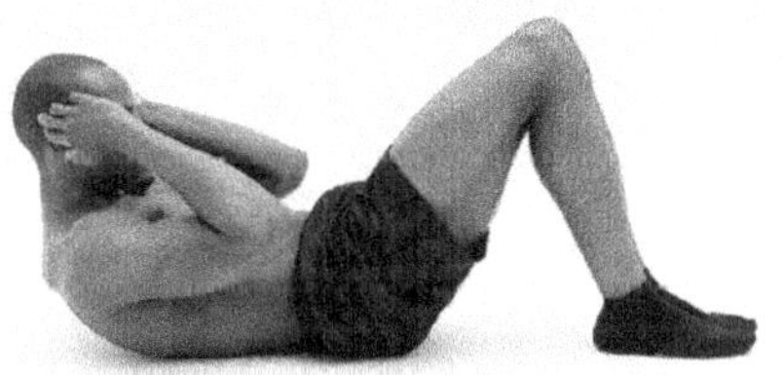

PLANK

The plank is a great core strength and stability exercise, and the chances are that you have already performed it before in some form or another.

Perform: 3-4 sets of 20-30 second hold times.

1. Get into regular push up position, but instead of placing your hands on the floor place your forearms flat against the floor straight out in front of you.

2. Balancing on your forearms and toes, raise your core until your body forms a straight line from your feet right through your knees, hips, and shoulders.

3. Hold this position for the allotted time or as long as possible to complete one set.

If you notice your back arching or your stomach sagging towards the ground, do your best to squeeze your abdominal muscles hard and keep your body in a straight line.

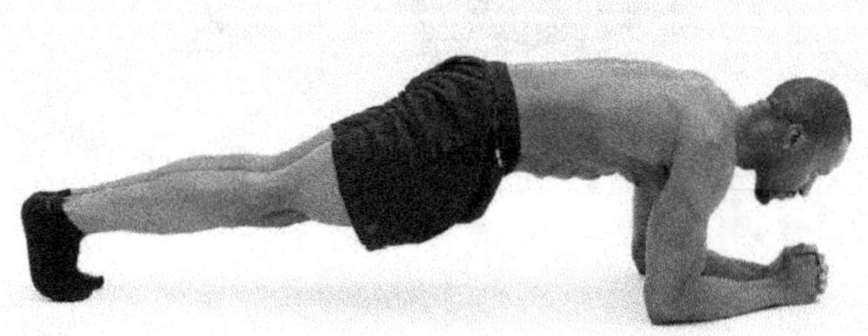

SIDE PLANK

This exercise will do for your obliques what regular the regular plank does for your abs, and is another great foundation exercise for your core.

Perform: 3-4 sets of 20-30 second hold times per side.

1. Lie on your side and support your upper bodyweight with one forearm placed on the ground at a 90-degree angle relative to the rest of your body.

2. With your bottom foot on its side, bring the other foot to rest on top of it.

3. Bring your hips up off the ground so your body forms a straight line.

4. Hold this position for allotted time or as long as possible to complete one set.

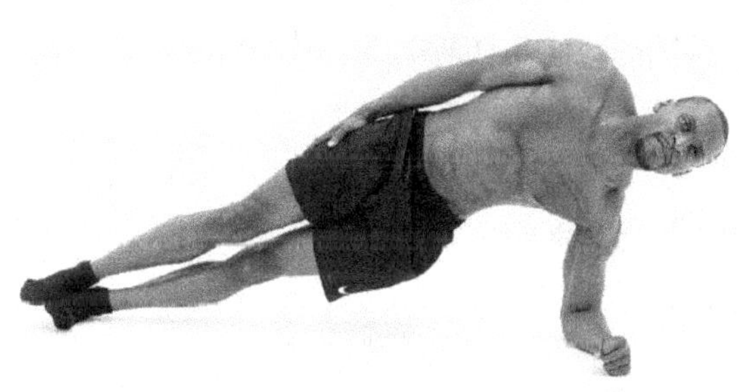

V-UP

Once you've nailed the previous exercises you can really test your core strength and stability with v-ups. Focus the tension in your core and use a soft surface to start with.

Perform: 3-4 sets of 10-15 reps.

1. Lie on your back with your arms by your sides and legs stretched out straight in front of you, feet slightly raised.

2. Lift your upper body off the ground while simultaneously bending your knees and bringing them up towards your chest. Keeping your arms and spine straight, aiming to move your hands past your knees.

3. When you have reached as far as possible, reverse the movement to complete one rep and go straight into the next.

Super important: With exercises such as this it is imperative that you make a conscious effort to concentrate the tension in your target muscles, i.e. the core.

Beginners have a tendency to lurch forward or lead with their neck, which not only completely defeats the purpose of the exercise, but also puts you at risk of injury.

If you find your neck getting sore it is a telltale sign that you are using improper form or that your core is not yet strong enough to perform this exercise.

In this case, first try correcting your form. If you're still not quite getting it, go back to the previous exercises to strengthen your core before coming back to this.

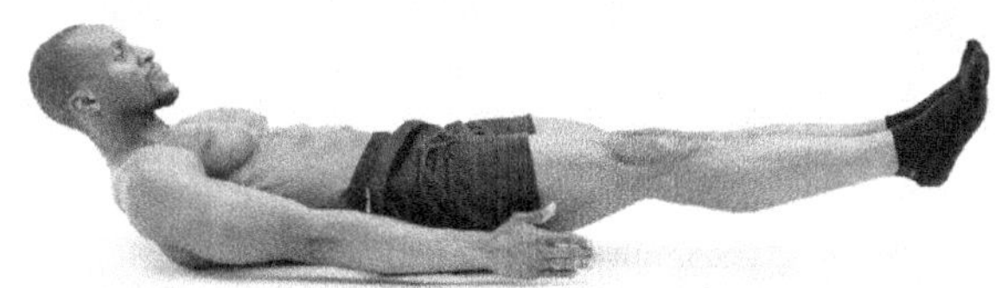

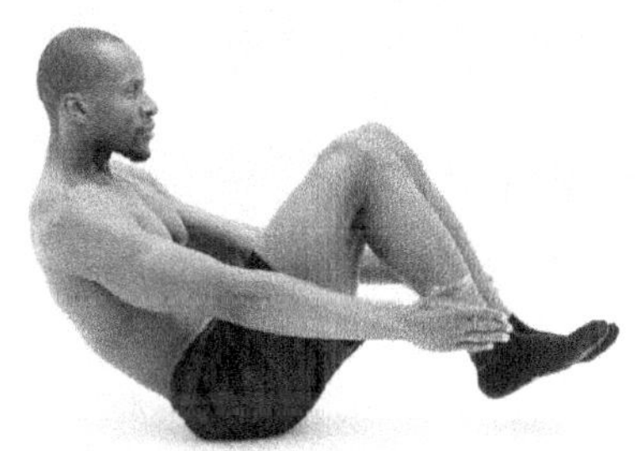

LYING LEG RAISES

This movement will target those hard to reach lower abdominal muscles, essential for core strength and good posture.

Perform: 3-4 sets of 15-20 reps.

1. Lie flat on your back with your legs stretched out in front of you, arms by your sides.

2. Keeping your upper body and lower back rooted to the floor and your legs straight, raise your legs to a 90-degree angle, or as high as you can with proper form.

3. Once you have reached the top position, reverse the movement to complete one repetition.

NB: Avoid touching your feet on the ground at the end of each rep. Maintaining core tension is key to building strength and stability.

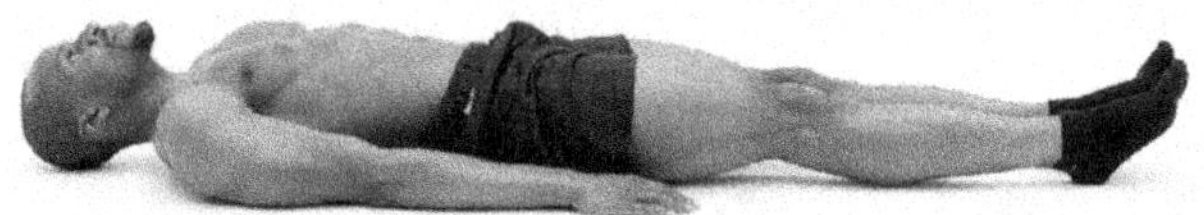

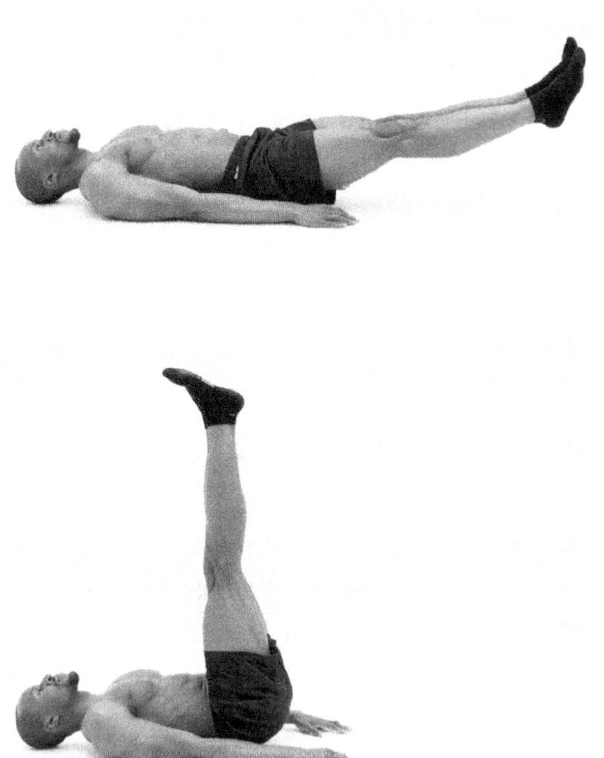

KNEE RAISES

Once you are comfortable with floor core exercises, head on over to a dip station or pull-up bar for a different kind of challenge.

Perform: 3-4 sets of 15-20 reps.

You will need: dip station / pull-up bar.

1. Grab the bar with an overhand grip and hang freely.

2. Bend your knees and draw your legs up towards your chest, contracting your core hard and focusing all the tension on the target muscles.

3. Return your legs to the starting position to complete one repetition. Make sure you are using your core and not momentum to achieve this movement.

Variation: If you don't have access to the equipment shown, you can use a dip station or captain's chair instead.

NB: It's not just your core that can tire during exercises like this. You might find your grip giving out, or your thighs burning up, for example.

This is your body's way of telling you that you have weak links somewhere in the chain. The good news is that with calisthenics you are almost always working more than one muscle group.

So, you will find that while you are doing knee raises to build a strong core, you are also generating forearm gains or hip flexibility, among other things.

Just don't forget that proper form is everything; if another area of your body is holding you back, make a note to work harder on that instead of cheating your way through.

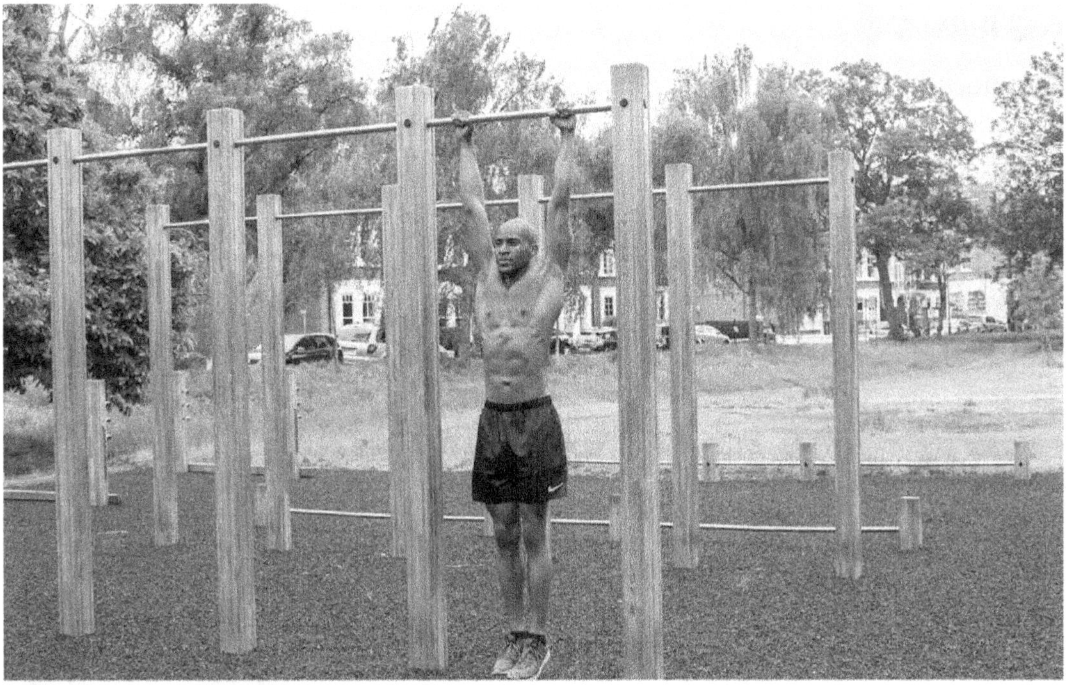

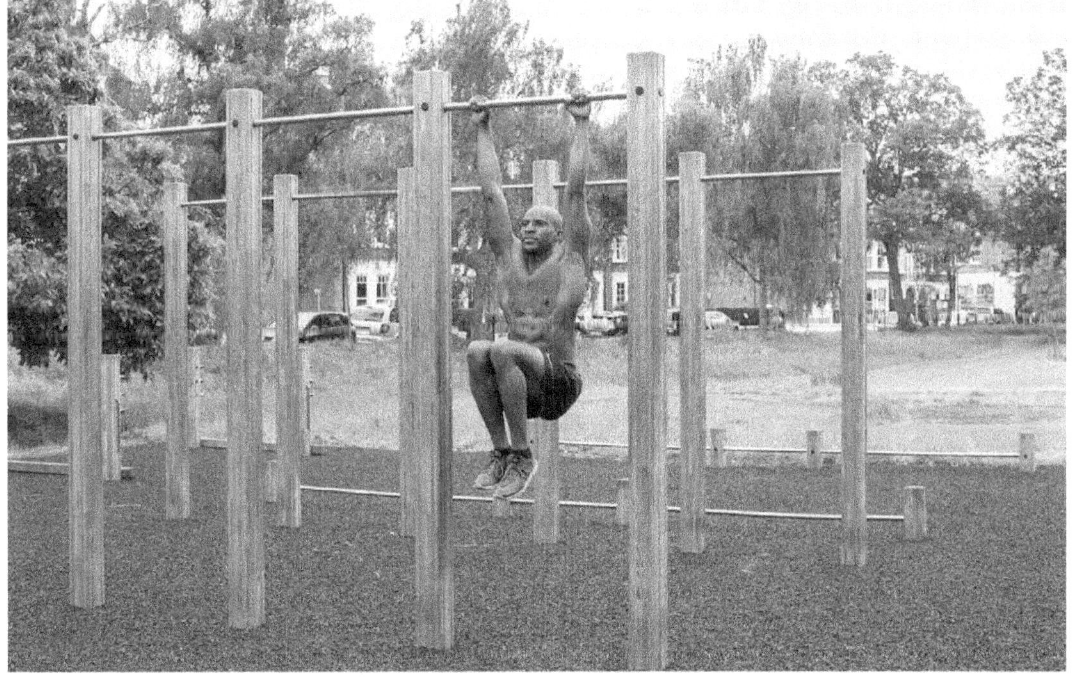

LEG RAISES

The natural progression from knee raises is to keep your legs straight and perform a similar movement, reaching up as high as you can without sacrificing form.

Perform: 3-4 sets of 10-15 reps.

You will need: a pull-up bar.

1. Grasp the bar with an overhand grip and let your legs hang straight down.

2. Using your core and not momentum, aim to bring your feet all the way up to your hands, keeping your legs straight throughout the movement.

3. Bring your legs back down to the start position to complete one rep.

NB: If you can't complete this range of movement, raise your legs as high as possible and increase the distance over time. The goal is to use your core for the vast majority of the movement, so do not lean back to achieve this until you are right at the top. Start by trying to get your legs parallel to the ground without moving your upper body.

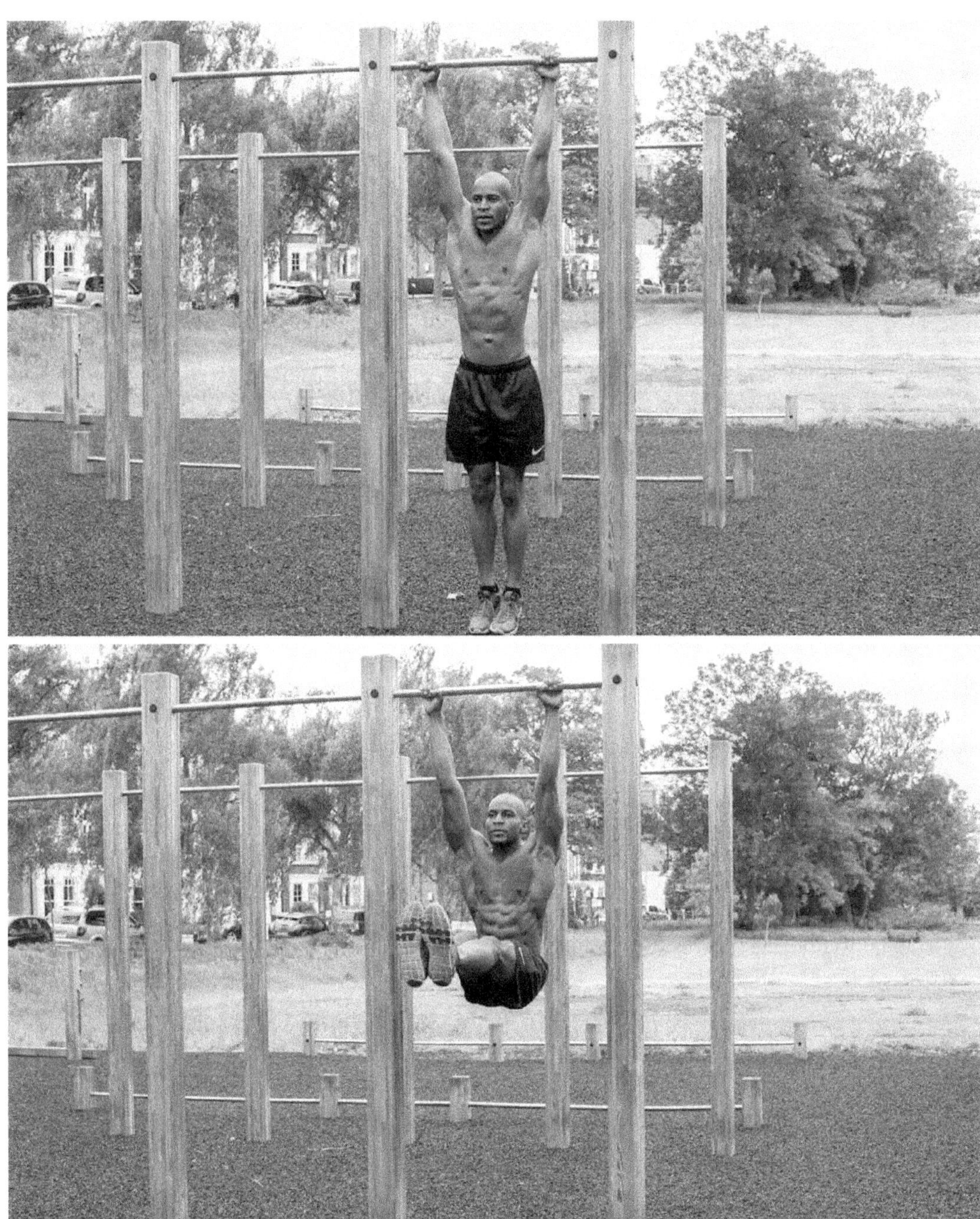

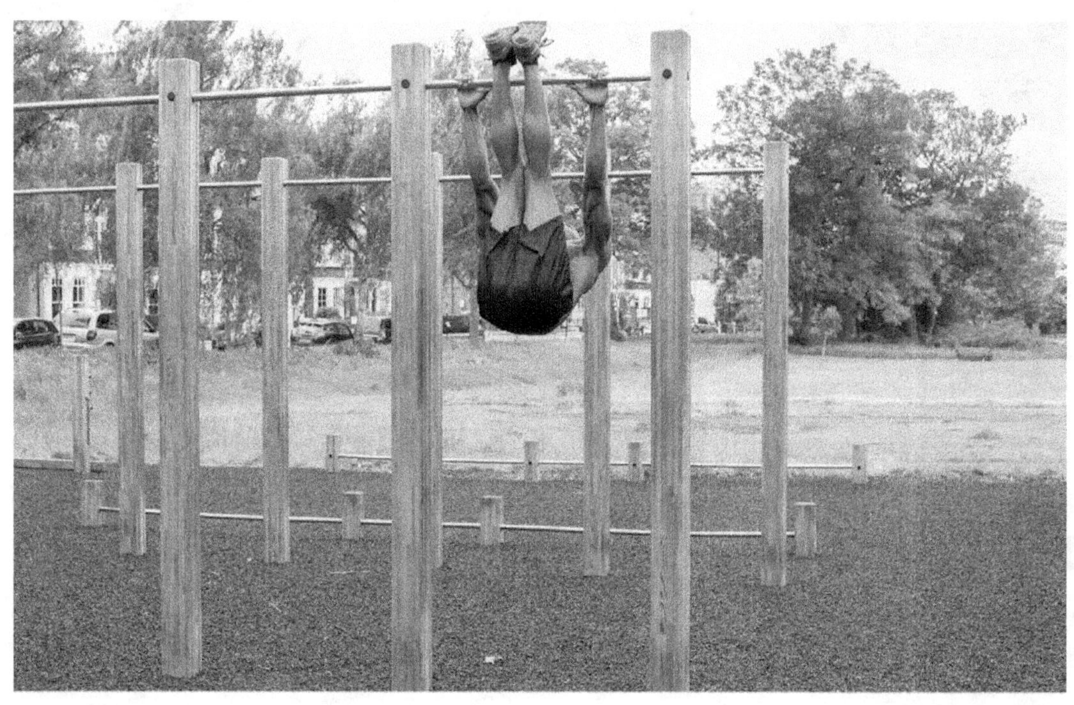

REAR ARCH

You will work your lower back with almost every core exercise you perform, but this is the first one we will cover which actually targets this area specifically.

Perform: 3-4 sets of 8-10 second hold times.

1. Lie down on your front and place your fingertips against your temples just as you did during sit-ups.

2. Aiming to keep your hips rooted to the floor, contract the muscles in your lower back and raise both your head and feet up as if you were trying to make them meet behind your back.

3. Hold for allotted time and then return to starting position to complete one rep.

Variations:

• When you have achieved your set / hold time gradually increase the hold time to keep improving.

• Try extending your arms out straight in front to make the exercise more difficult.

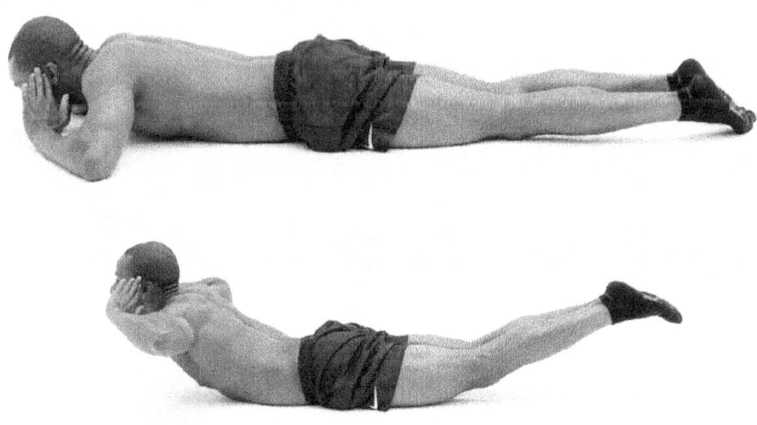

REAR SUPPORT

This one will really engage your core muscles while opening up your hip flexors to help you perform the lower body stuff to come.

Perform: 3-4 sets of 10-15 second hold times.

1. Sit on the ground with your legs straight out in front of you and your hands by your sides, fingers facing backwards.

2. Balancing on your hands and heels, push your hips up and try to align your whole body from ankles to shoulders.

3. Hold this position for as long as is possible to complete one set. As with all similar exercises, gradually increase the hold time to improve your strength and resistance.

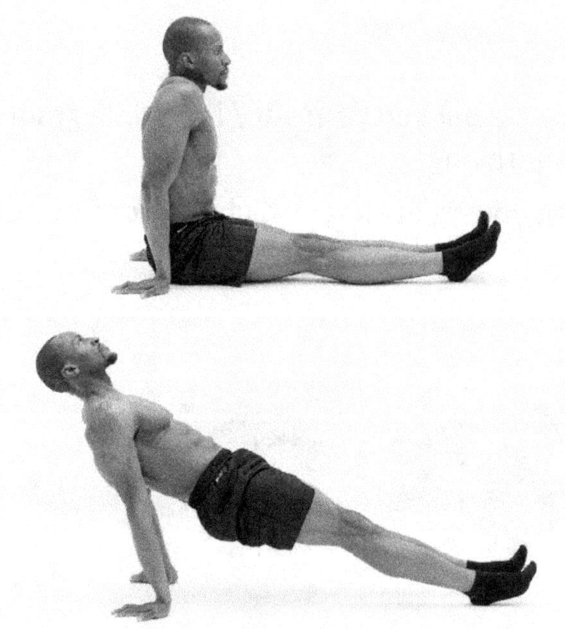

LOWER BODY

Now that we've covered upper body and core exercises it's time to move on to the lower body. There is a misconception that lower body is somehow less important when training calisthenics and that it is overlooked in favor of the other muscle groups, but if you want your body to work in perfect unison then you need to respect every area.

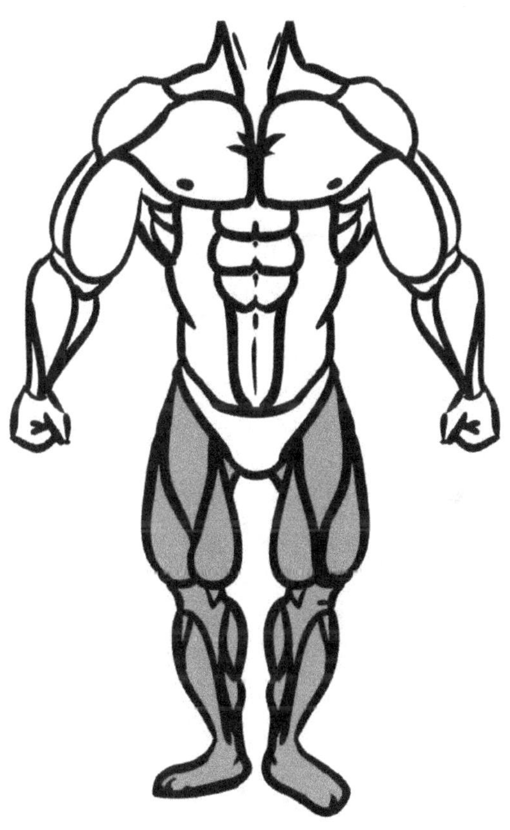

FUNDAMENTALS

We recommend adding these fundamental exercises to your lower body workout. As always, work through them progressively and only move on when you are completely competent in performing the easier exercises. Ready? Set? Then let's get straight to it!

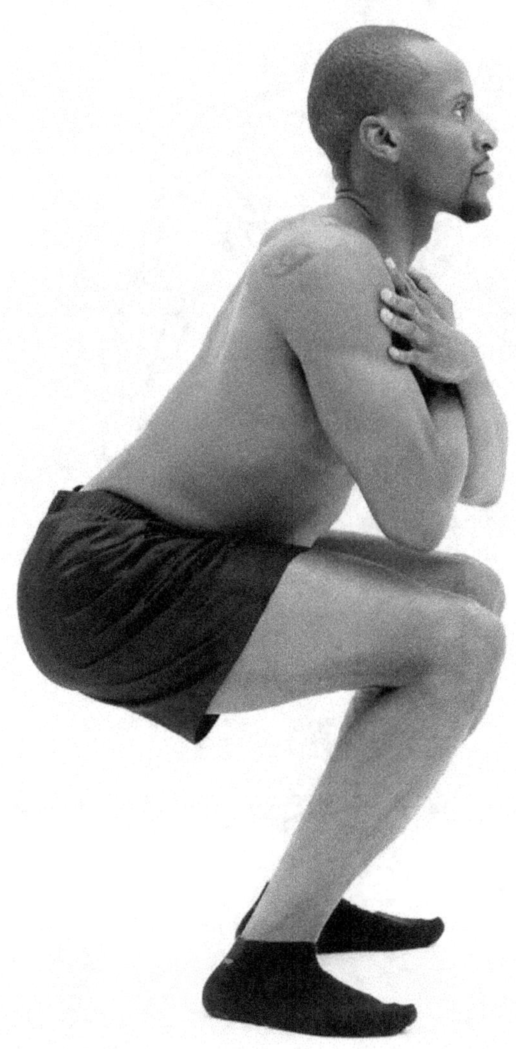

CALF RAISES

This is a staple exercise for your lower legs and will test your calves severely.

Perform: 4-5 sets of 20-30 reps.

1. Stand with your feet approximately shoulder width apart, arms by your sides.

2. Contract your calves and push yourself up to stand on your toes.

3. Lower yourself back down to the starting position in a steady, controlled movement to complete one rep.

Variation: Perform this exercise while crouched down for a different kind of challenge.

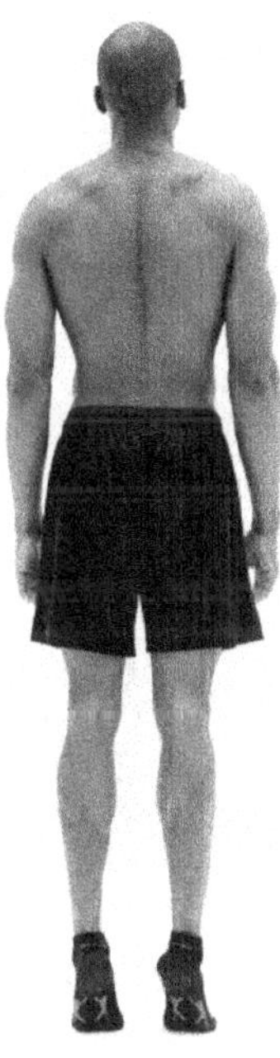

BRIDGE

The bridge is a fairly simple exercise designed to target your glutes and lower body.

Perform: 3-4 sets of 20-30 second holds.

1. Lay on your back with your arms by your sides, knees bent at around 90 degrees and feet rooted flat to the floor.

2. Keeping your upper body planted, raise your hips and try to align them with your knees and shoulders.

3. Hold this position for as long as possible before returning to the start position to complete one rep.

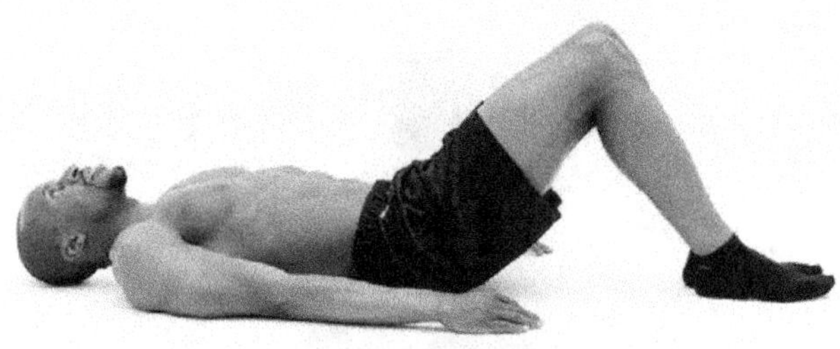

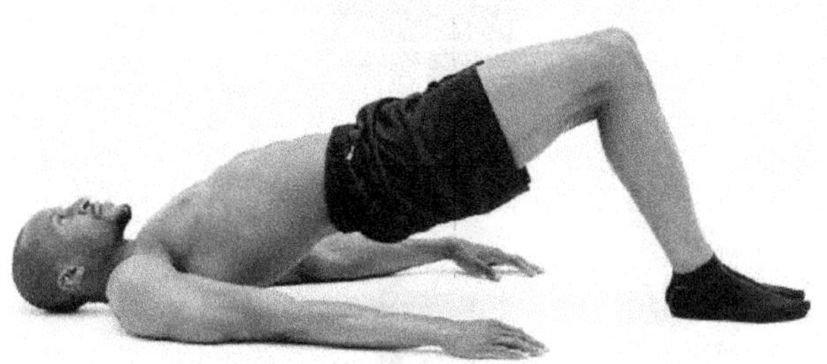

SQUATS

Everybody's heard of them and, believe it or not, everybody's done them in some form or another. Whether you've performed them on a rack at the gym, or simply by bending down to pick up the laundry, this movement should be familiar to one and all.

The humble squat works your quads, hips, glutes, hamstrings, adductors and lower back, making it a fundamental movement for anyone wanting to gain strength and power.

Perform: 4-5 sets of 10-15 reps.

1. Stand with your feet approximately shoulder width apart and toes at an angle that is comfortable for you.

2. Fold your arms across your chest or extend them out in front of you if you need more help with balance.

3. Keeping your feet firmly rooted, your arms in position and your spine straight, bend your knees and push your hips backwards whilst lowering to the ground. Open your knees out a little to make room if required.

4. Lower your hips as far as possible without actually sitting. In line with your knees or anywhere past this point is fine.

5. Once you have reached this position, drive from your glutes and quads to bring your hips back up to the starting position to complete one rep.

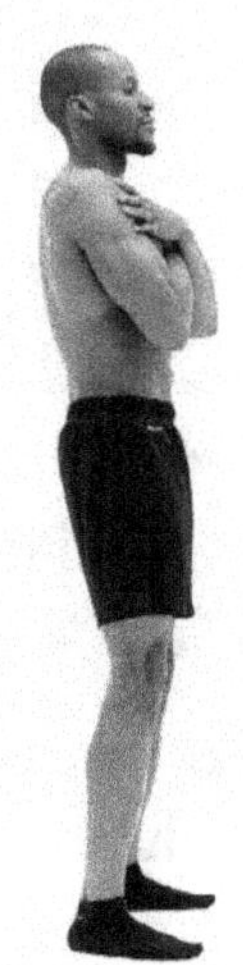

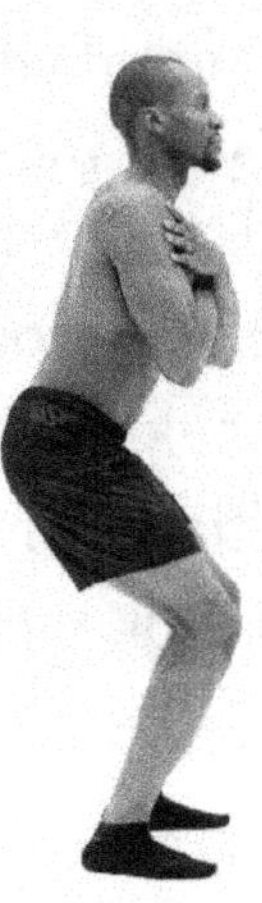

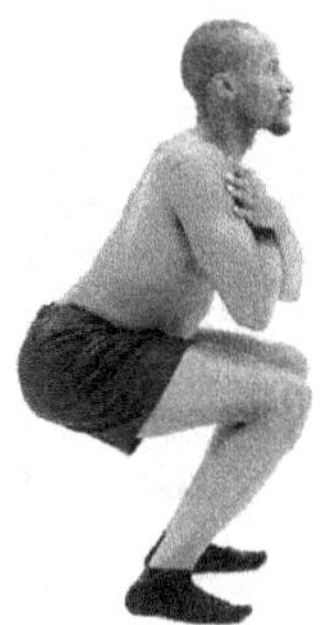

LUNGES

It's time to get a bit more mobile and develop some more functional strength in your lower body. These ones will burn up your quads and glutes in particular.

Perform: 3-4 sets of 10-15 reps per leg.

1. Stand with your feet approximately shoulder width apart, arms by your sides.

2. Keeping one foot rooted to the ground, take a step forward with the other.

3. In one seamless movement and keeping your upper body as upright as possible, plant your front foot on the ground and bend both knees until the knee of your back leg comes close to the floor.

4. From here drive back to the starting position by pushing hard with your front leg. This completes one repetition, so you'll then need to switch legs and repeat the exercise.

Variations:

• Make this a seamless movement by 'walking' continuously into the next reps.

• Hold weights to increase the load on your muscles.

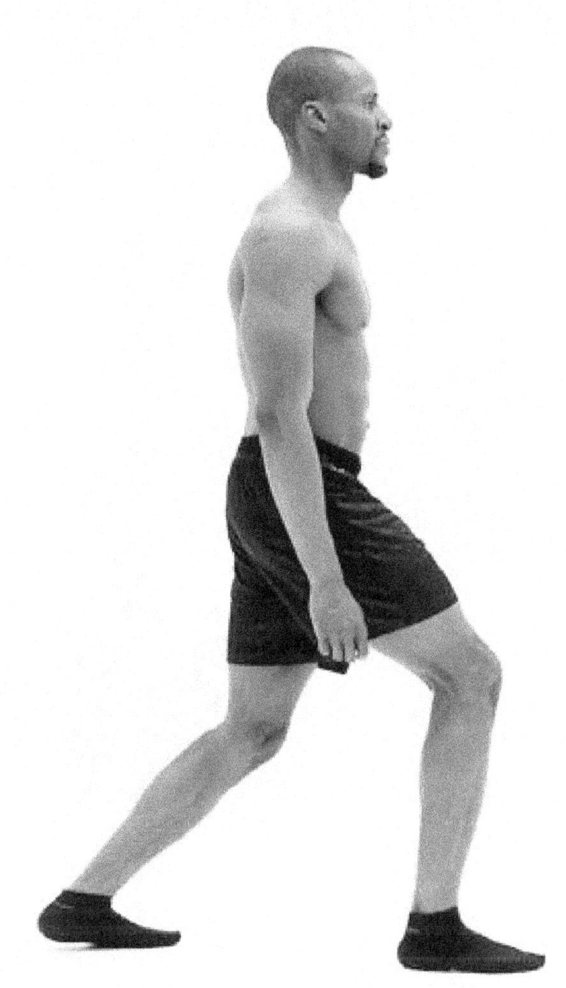

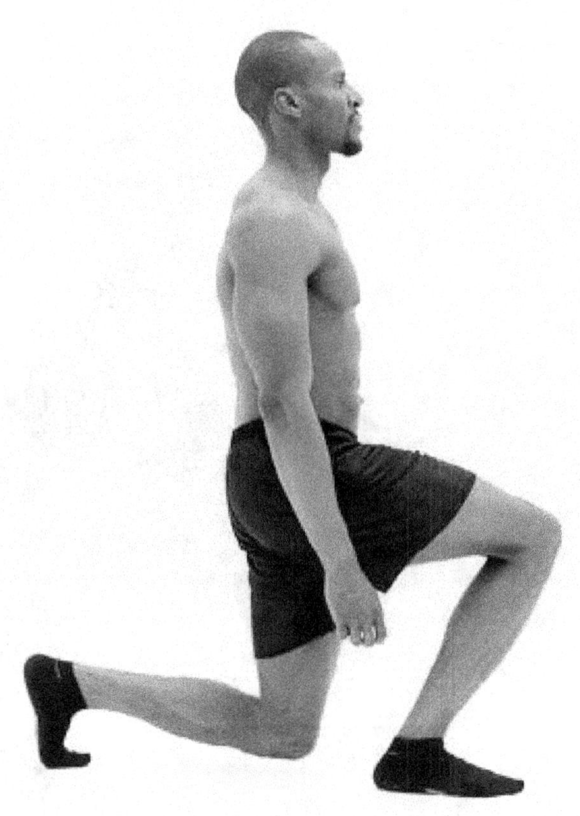

BODYWEIGHT DEADLIFT

The deadlift is a fundamental exercise right across the fitness community and will help build lower body strength while stabilizing your core.

Perform: 3-4 sets of 8-12 reps.

1. Stand up straight, arms hanging by your sides, ready to begin the exercise.

2. Bend down, maintaining a straight back and sticking your glutes out behind you.

3. Reach down as far as is comfortable with the correct form, and then reverse the movement to complete one rep.

NB: For many people, flexibility is a greater barrier to achieving this exercise than strength. If that is the case for you, identify the tight areas using the body map near the front of this book, and go back through the suggested mobility and flexibility exercises.

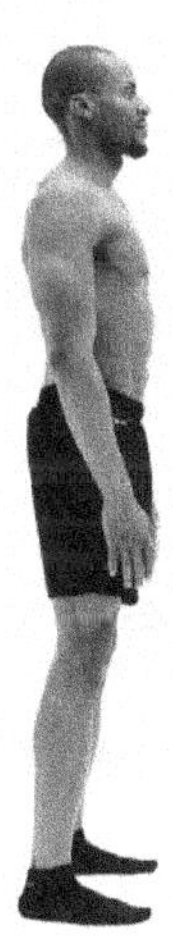

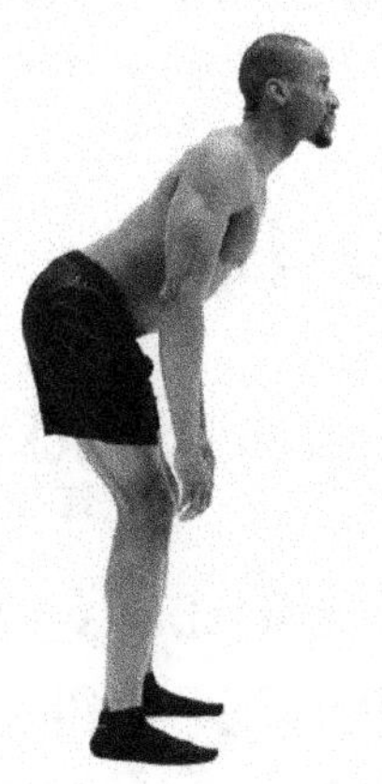

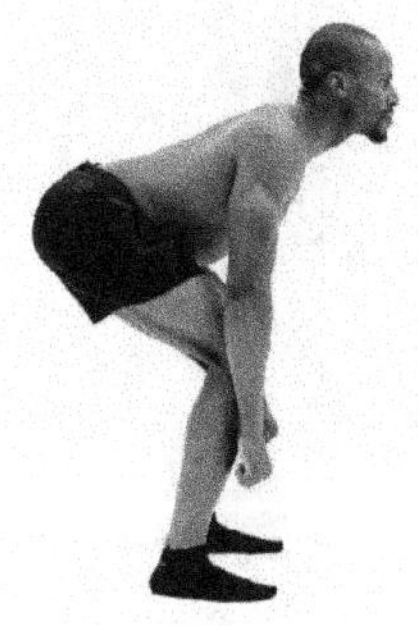

"Champions aren't made in gyms. Champions are made from something they have deep inside them — a desire, a dream, a vision. They have to have last-minute stamina, they have to be a little

faster, they have to have the skill and the will. But the will must be stronger than the skill."

Muhammad Ali

6. CARDIO & CONDITIONING

Welcome to HELL! Your final task is to power through the fire and come out the other side keeled over, dripping in sweat, but completely and utterly satisfied that you left absolutely NOTHING on the table.

Yes, this is a book focused on calisthenics, but it would be criminal to omit cardiovascular exercise and general conditioning, as this is the gateway to a truly SUPERHUMAN body. By performing these exercises you will condition your body to be able to work harder and go longer, thereby allowing you to compound your results exponentially.

You will also turn your body into a fat burning furnace, blasting belly fat and allowing your finely tuned muscles to come to the fore. For building popping six-pack abs and obliques in particular, this is non-negotiable. We are truly into no pain, no gain territory!

Remember, the name of the game here is not slow and steady; conditioning is all about intensity. Throw everything you have at the following exercises – if your heart isn't pounding, if you're not covered in sweat, then you're not training hard enough!

Don't be one of those people who sits idly on a bike, scrolling through their Facebook feed and working out their thumbs more than the rest of their body. And you better not skip it altogether either, because this guide comes as a package, just like your body.

If you're still in doubt as to the benefits of cardio and conditioning, here's a quick recap:

1. INCREASE METABOLISM: This becomes increasingly important as the years go by and your metabolism slows down. In order to achieve a peak state of being, use cardio to keep your metabolism running at full throttle!

2. KEEP YOUR HEART HEALTHY: Your heart just so happens to be the muscle that runs the entire show, and cardiovascular exercise is how you give it a workout. Look after your ticker, and it will look after you!

3. IMPROVE RECOVERY TIME: A spot of cardio after a heavy session can reduce your DOMS (Delayed Onset of Muscle Soreness) and rush healing, oxygen rich blood to the muscle tissues. Translation: you can get back in the game quicker!

4. BURN FAT AND LOOK AWESOME: The simple fact of the matter is that you will never burn that stubborn fat and achieve your dream body without cardio. So, how about we just quit all this jibber jabber and knock it out of the park!

INTERVAL SPRINTS

Welcome to the pinnacle of cardio and conditioning exercises. Sprinting will get your heart pounding and your muscles working overtime to deliver INSANE results.

Super important: We must say it, but it truly is super important. Please, never perform cardiovascular activity without having had a thorough physical. Better safe than sorry.

Perform: 5-10 sets of 10-15 second bursts.

1. Take up the traditional starting position for a sprint, ready to spring off from one foot. If you are on a treadmill or free running, prepare to increase the speed.

2. With a powerful burst, break into as fast a sprint as you possibly can and do not stop until you reach your target to complete 1 set.

3. Rest for 30 secs or so and then go again. In this case, jogging can be a form of rest!

NB: Going from zero to everything can be risky, so make double sure that you have properly warmed up before launching into this kind of activity.

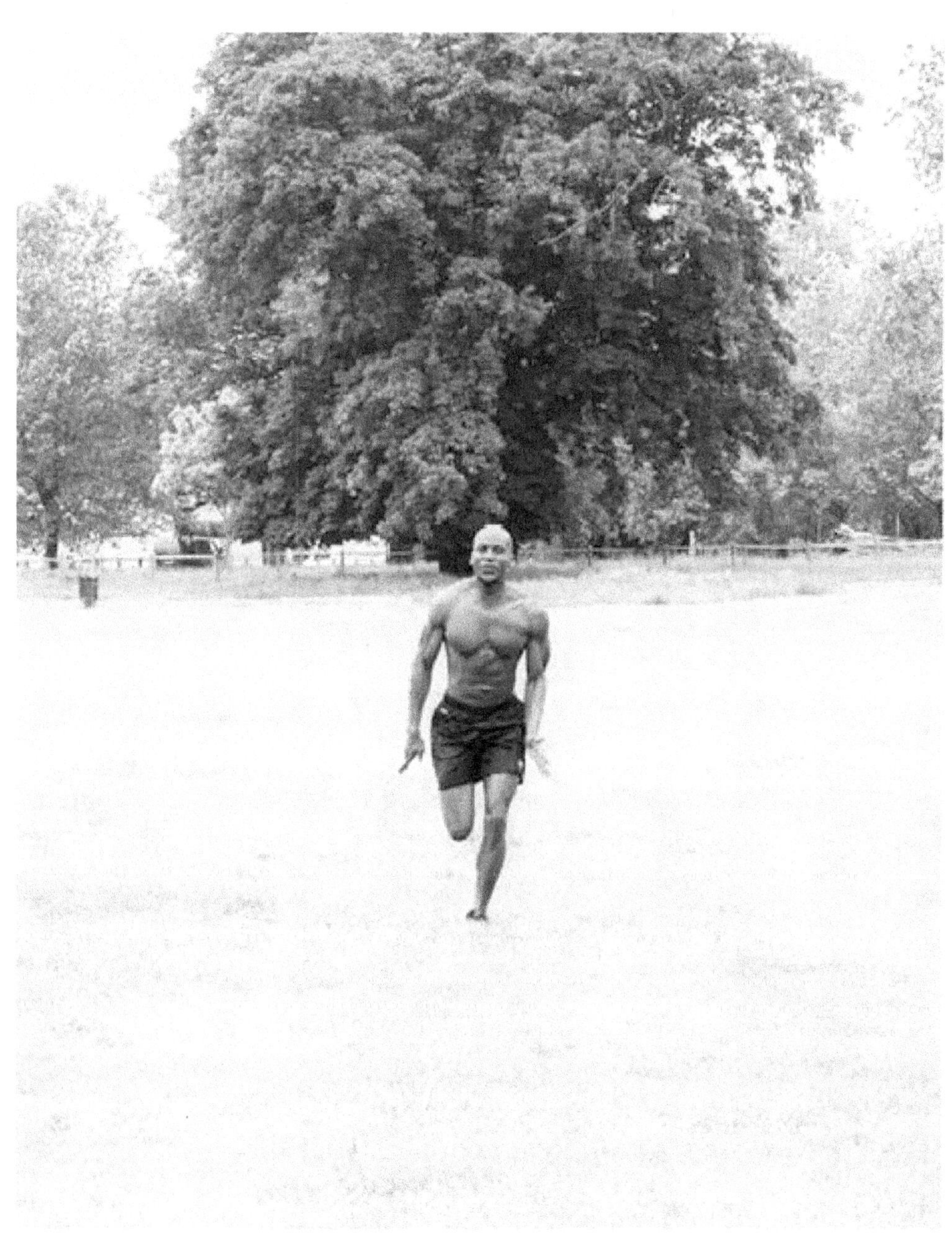

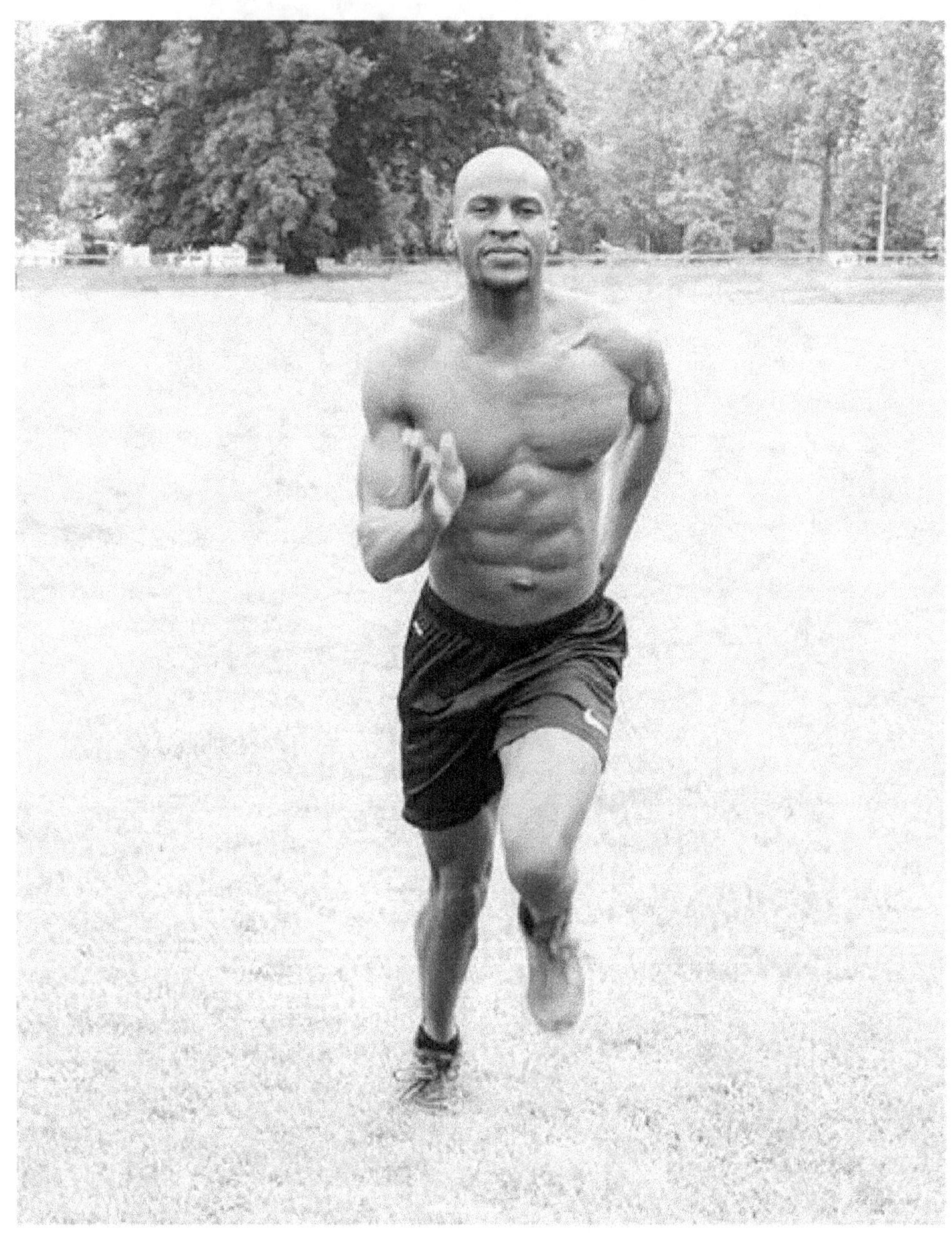

JUMPING SQUAT

We covered the squat earlier on so you should be used to performing this movement in some capacity already, but it's now time to explore a more intense alternative.

Perform: 3-4 sets of 20-30 reps.

1. Take up the same starting position as regular squats, standing with your feet shoulder width apart.

2. Squat down as you would for regular squats.

3. Launch yourself into the air as high as possible.

4. Upon landing, bend your knees to absorb the impact and compete one rep, using the momentum generated to launch straight into the next rep.

Remember: You can always mix things up by working out against the clock instead of using a sets and reps system.

A mixture of the two, i.e. seeing how may reps you can perform in a certain amount of time, can be particularly effective when training cardio.

It's useful to have a training buddy when it comes to this kind of exercise, as it is pretty darn exhausting and you might find their support helps you find the strength to rock out that final rep.

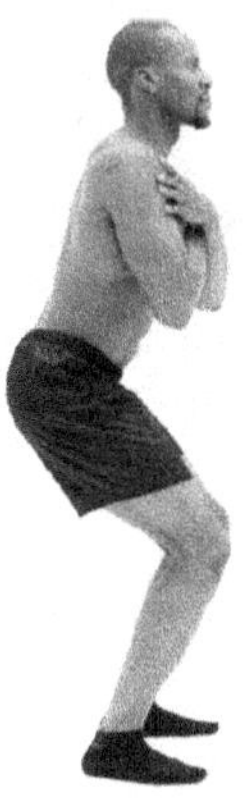

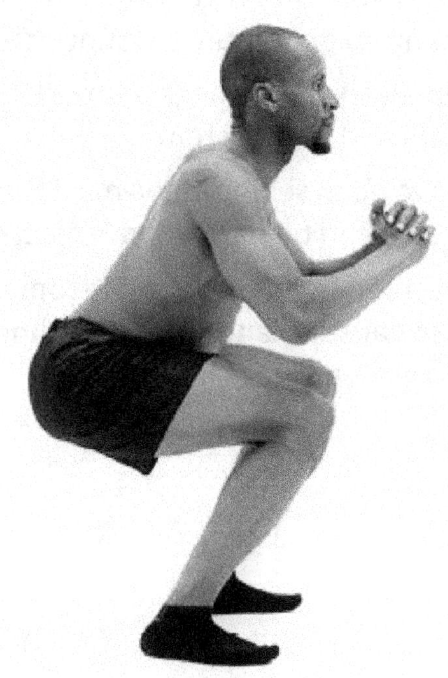

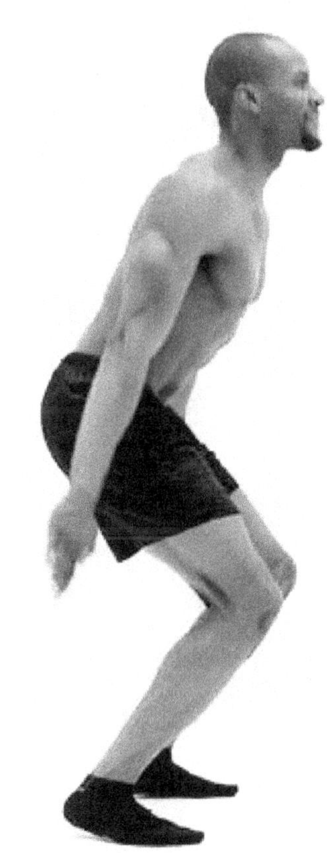

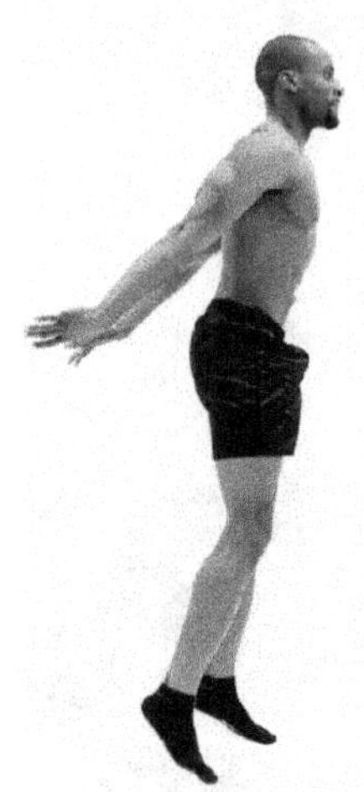

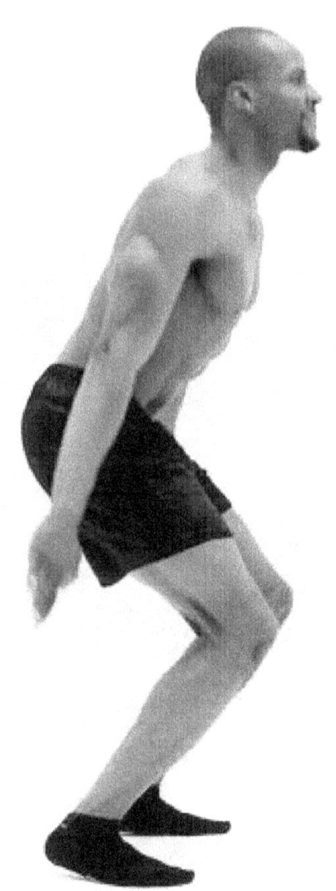

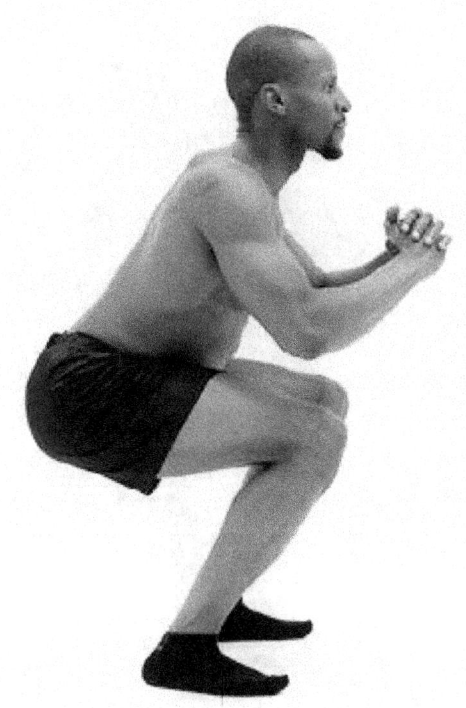

SQUAT THRUST

We're getting a little more advanced now, but most people should still be comfortable with this exercise, with a little practice.

You'll soon notice that you are also getting a pretty decent full body workout in addition to your cardio hit. Embrace it. It's all part of become your best self.

Perform: 3-4 sets of 20-30 reps.

1. Squat down on your toes with your knees tucked against your chest and palms flat on floor in front of your feet.

2. Keeping your palms rooted, spring your feet off the ground and propel them backwards so you effectively land in the push-up position.

3. Reverse the movement, springing your feet back into the starting position to complete one repetition.

NB: If you've just performed this exercise for the first time, you will realize that it's more than just a cardio hit.

The squat thrust also calls upon your arms for support, your lower body for that explosive push off, and above all your core for hauling yourself into position.

For those who straight up hate cardio, there is at least some solace to be had in the knowledge that you are working hard on those other key areas, too!

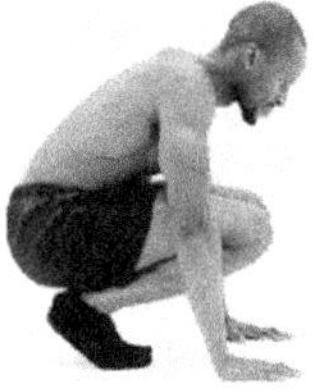

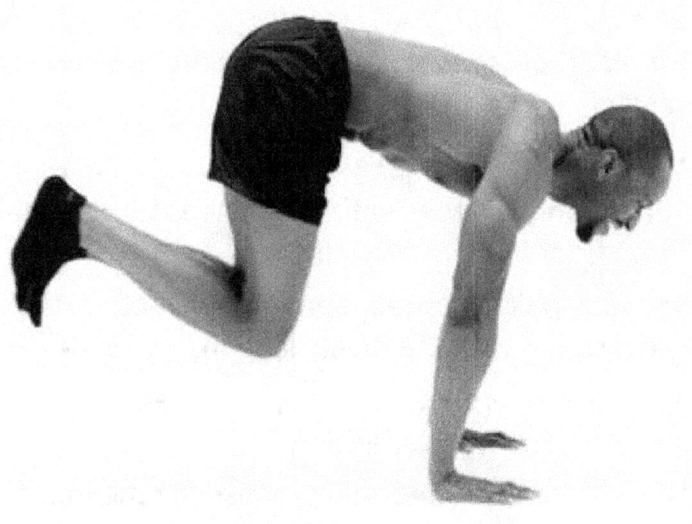

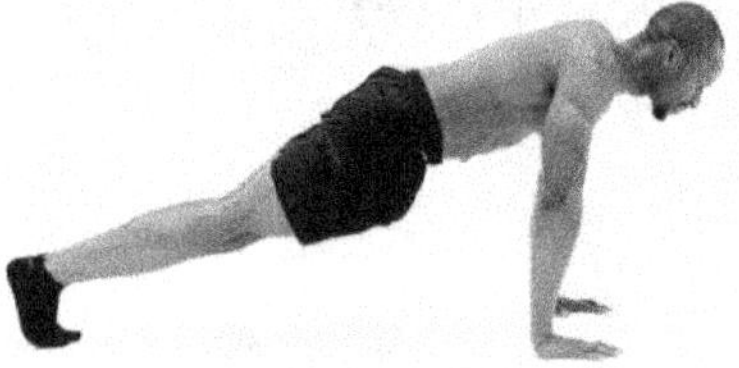

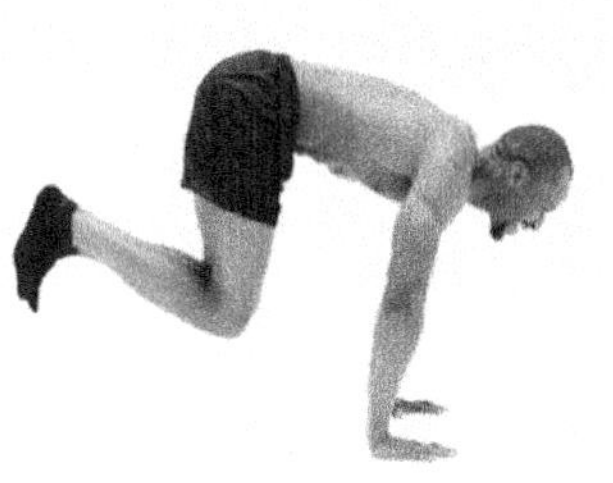

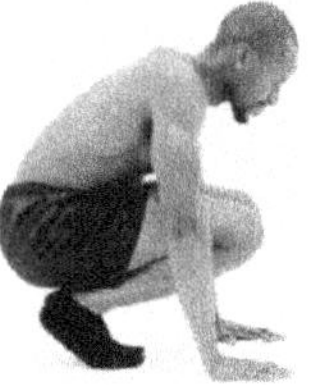

MOUNTAIN CLIMBERS

Essentially a variation on the squat thrust, the mountain climber is an excellent addition to your cardio and conditioning repertoire.

Perform: 3-4 sets of 20-30 reps.

1. Take up the push-up position, except this time bring one foot right up until it's just behind your hands.

2. Spring your feet into the air and switch their positions, bringing the front one to the back and vice versa.

3. Reverse the action to bring your legs back to starting position to complete one rep. You can fire straight into the next rep from here.

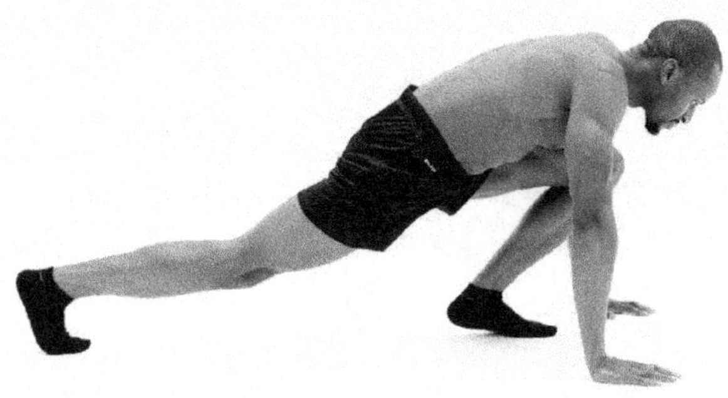

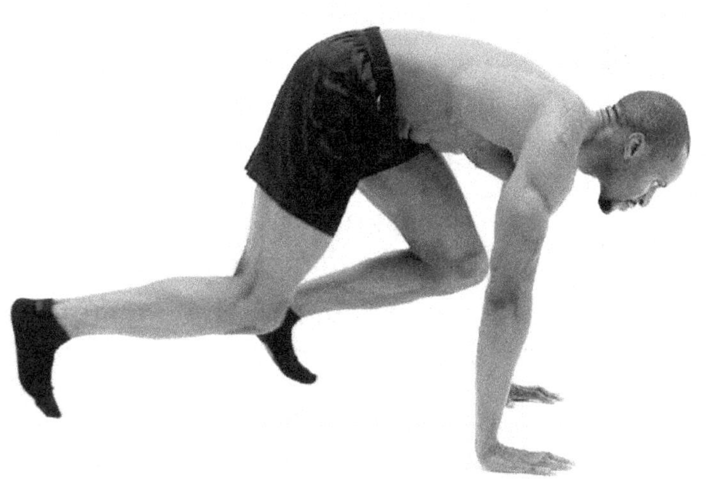

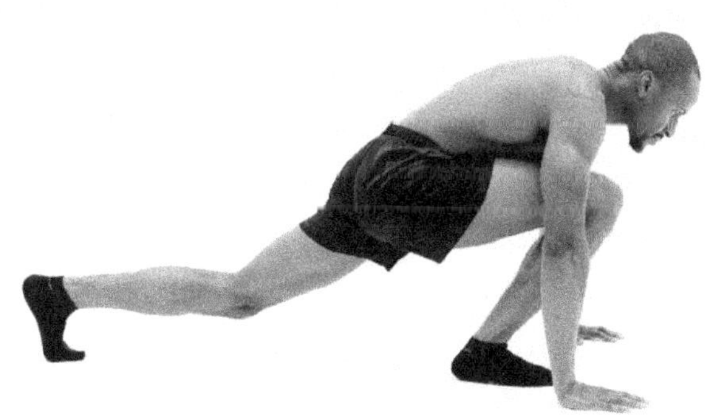

JUMPING LUNGE

Another variation on an exercise we've already covered, the jumping lunge is a great way to condition your lower body at the same time as getting an intense cardio hit.

Perform: 3-4 sets of 6-10 reps on each leg.

1. Take up the lunge position with one foot forward and both knees bent, the rear one close to the ground.

2. Jump into the air, aiming to get as much height as possible, and switch leg positions, bringing the front one to the back and vice versa.

3. Bend your knees upon landing to complete one repetition and use the momentum generated to go on and perform a full set.

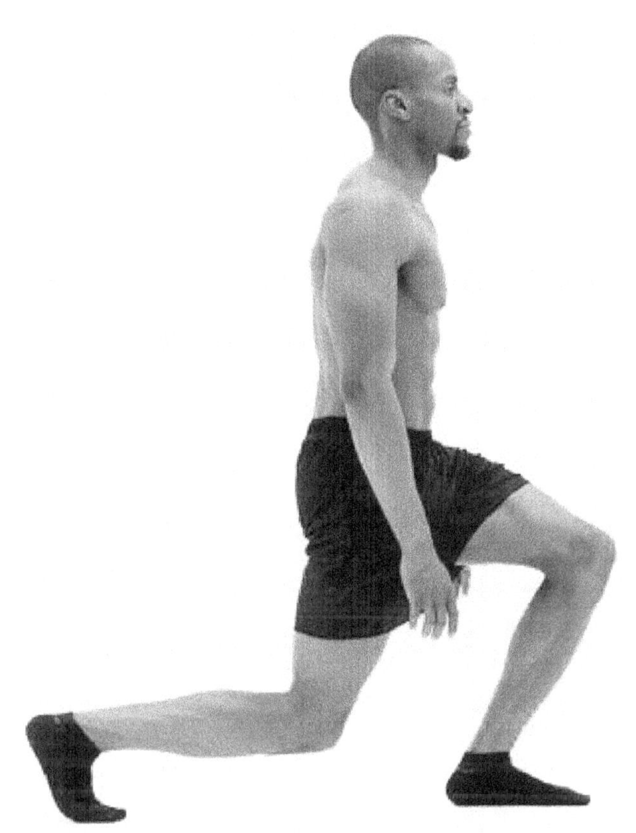

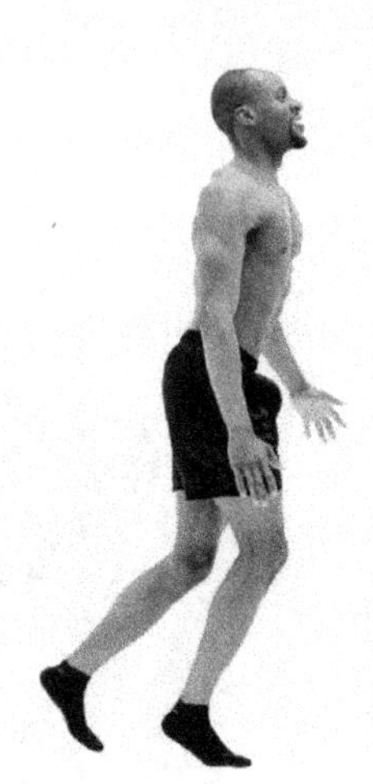

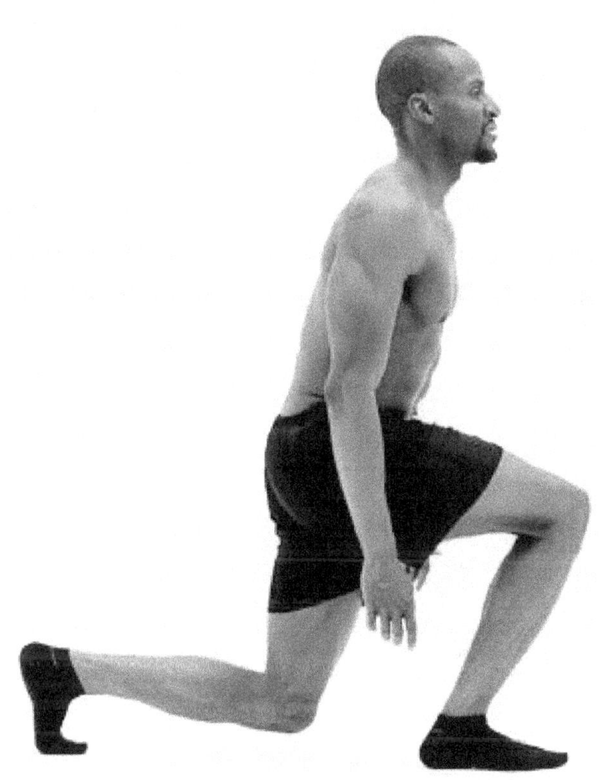

STAR JUMPS

Favored for its simplicity and famed for its effectiveness, the humble star jump is the staple of fitness regimes the world over. It is extremely likely that you have done this exercise before, but here's a reminder of how to complete it with proper form anyway.

Perform: 3-4 sets of 20-30 reps.

1. Stand up straight, feet together and arms by your sides.

2. Jump into the air stretching your arms and feet out to the sides.

3. Land with your feet wide apart and arms raised straight above your head.

4. Return to starting position by jumping up into the air again, bringing your feet back together and arms to your sides. You have now performed one repetition.

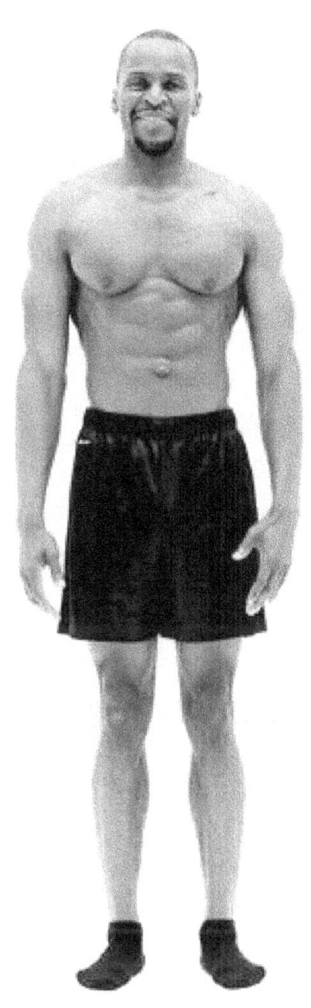

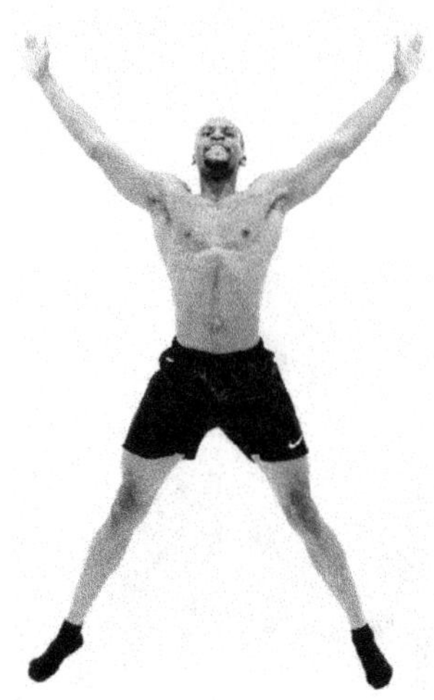

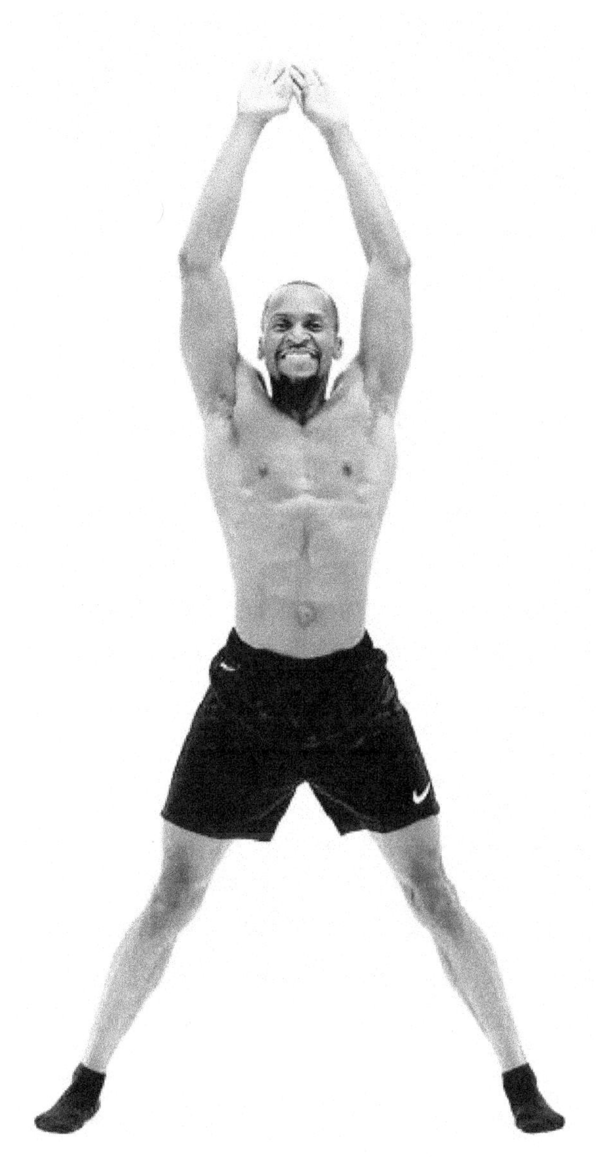

BURPEES

You are about to call upon every muscle sinew in your body to complete one of the most effective conditioning exercises known to man, so get warmed up and prepare for pain!

Perform: 3-4 sets of 10-20 reps.

1. Take up the squat thrust position, crouched down on your toes with your knees tucked against your chest and palms flat on floor in front of your feet.

2. Palms rooted, spring your feet into the air and thrust your legs backwards so you land in the push-up position.

3. Reverse this movement, springing your feet into the air again and landing back in the starting position.

4. Jump straight upwards as high as you can, bending your knees upon landing to reassume the position in step 1 to complete one rep.

Remember: Keep it moving with exercises like this. Pushing on through exhaustion is how progress is made. Never just go through the motions or quit as soon as the going gets tough!

You may find it particularly difficult to keep track of sets and reps when your heart is busy pumping oxygen to every extremity, so setting a timer and working to the clock is a great way to train if you're going solo.

If you have a training partner, have them count you down, and don't be afraid of a little competition. You might just bring the best out of each other.

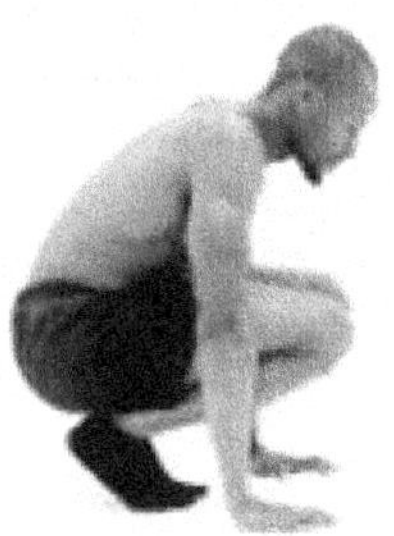

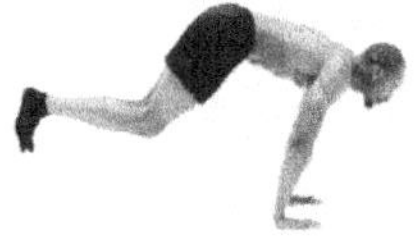

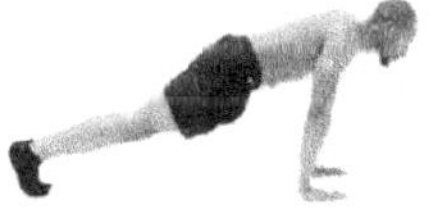

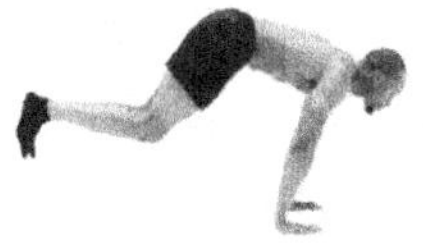

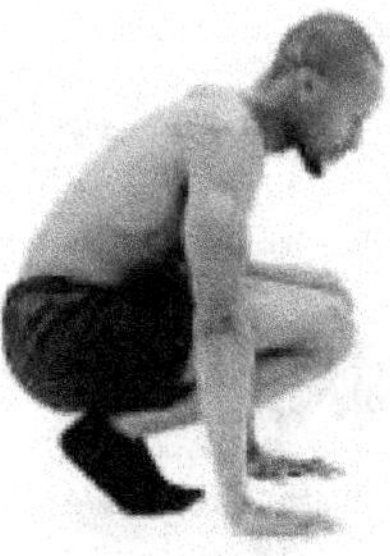

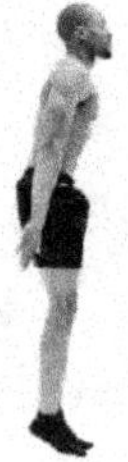

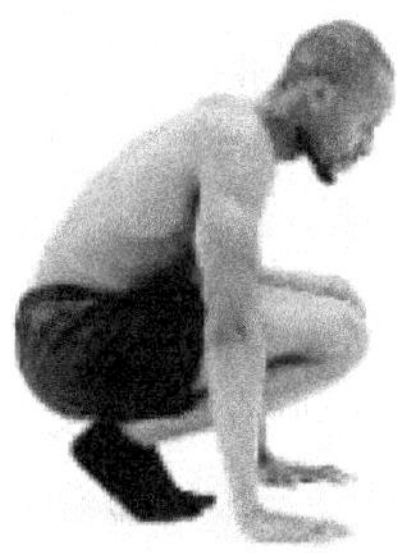

ADVANCED BURPEES

Essentially the same as the burpee, except we're tossing a push-up into the middle of each rep. Some call it the 'bastard', and you're about to find out why!

Perform: 3-4 sets of 10-20 reps.

1. Assume the same starting position as the burpee, crouched down, knees just behind your hands, braced for the punishment to come.

2. Now kick your feet back to push-up position as before.

3. Knock out 1 push-up.

4. When you are back at the top of the push-up position, kick your feet back to the crouched position.

5. Now jump straight up into the air, aiming for the moon!

6. Land back in the crouched position and go again.

Are you feeling the burn? If you said no, you're lying. But fear not, for we are about to draw this cardio and conditioning section to a close.

We have one more offering which is sure to attract some double takes out in public, but don't be afraid to go all in. After all, you get out exactly what you put in.

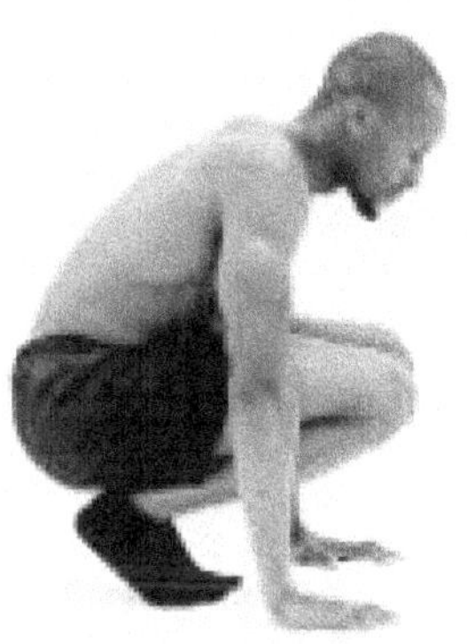

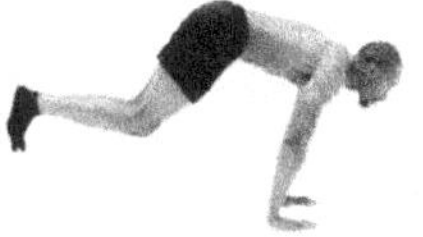

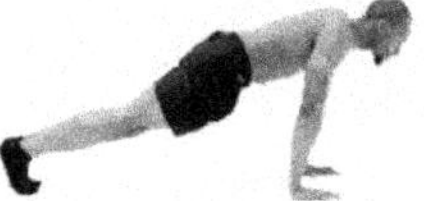

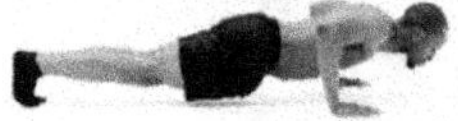

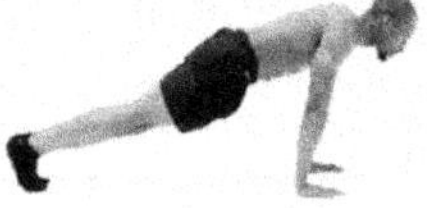

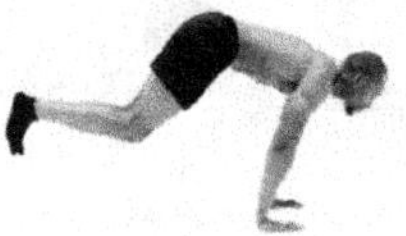

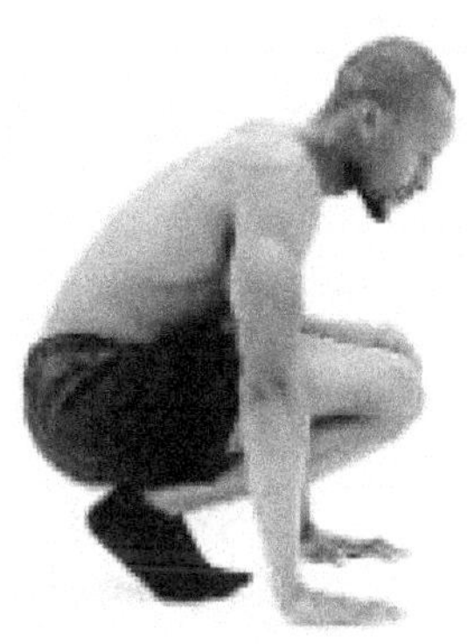

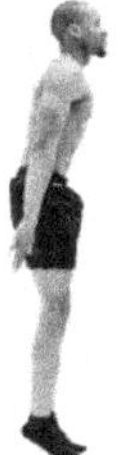

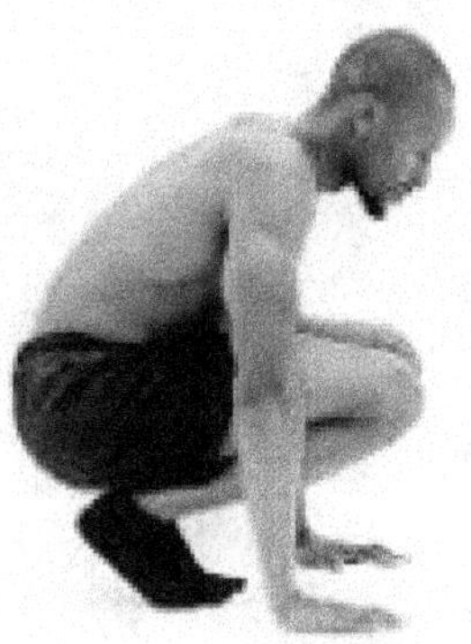

BEAR CRAWLS

This is another brutal conditioning exercise, but pain really does mean gain here so commit to completing it and you will see and feel the benefits.

Perform: 3-4 sets of 15-20 second crawls.

1. Take up the push-up position.

2. Place one hand forward, and bring the opposite foot forward too. Continue crawling like this, alternating your hands and legs, until you reach your threshold.

3. Repeat for allocated number of sets.

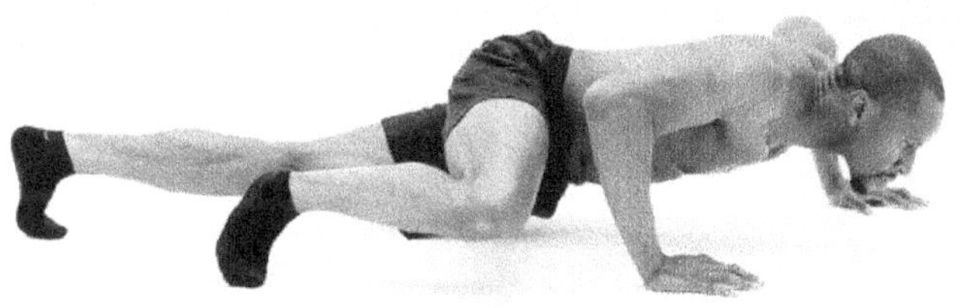

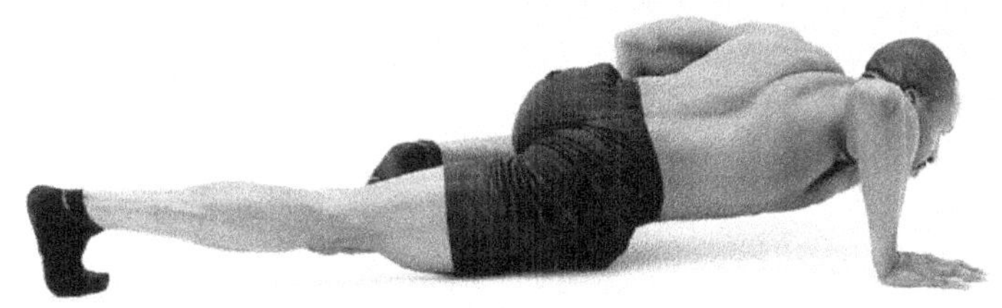

SKIPPING

Skipping is a great cardiovascular exercise that is often used for warming up or down as well as general fitness training.

Perform: 3-4 sets of 20-30 second bursts.

1. Grab your rope and swing it over your head.

2. From here you can either choose to jump both feet over the rope, or skip one foot at a time. If you're feeling really fancy, you can even do a criss cross.

Variation: Pick up a weighted rope for a greater challenge.

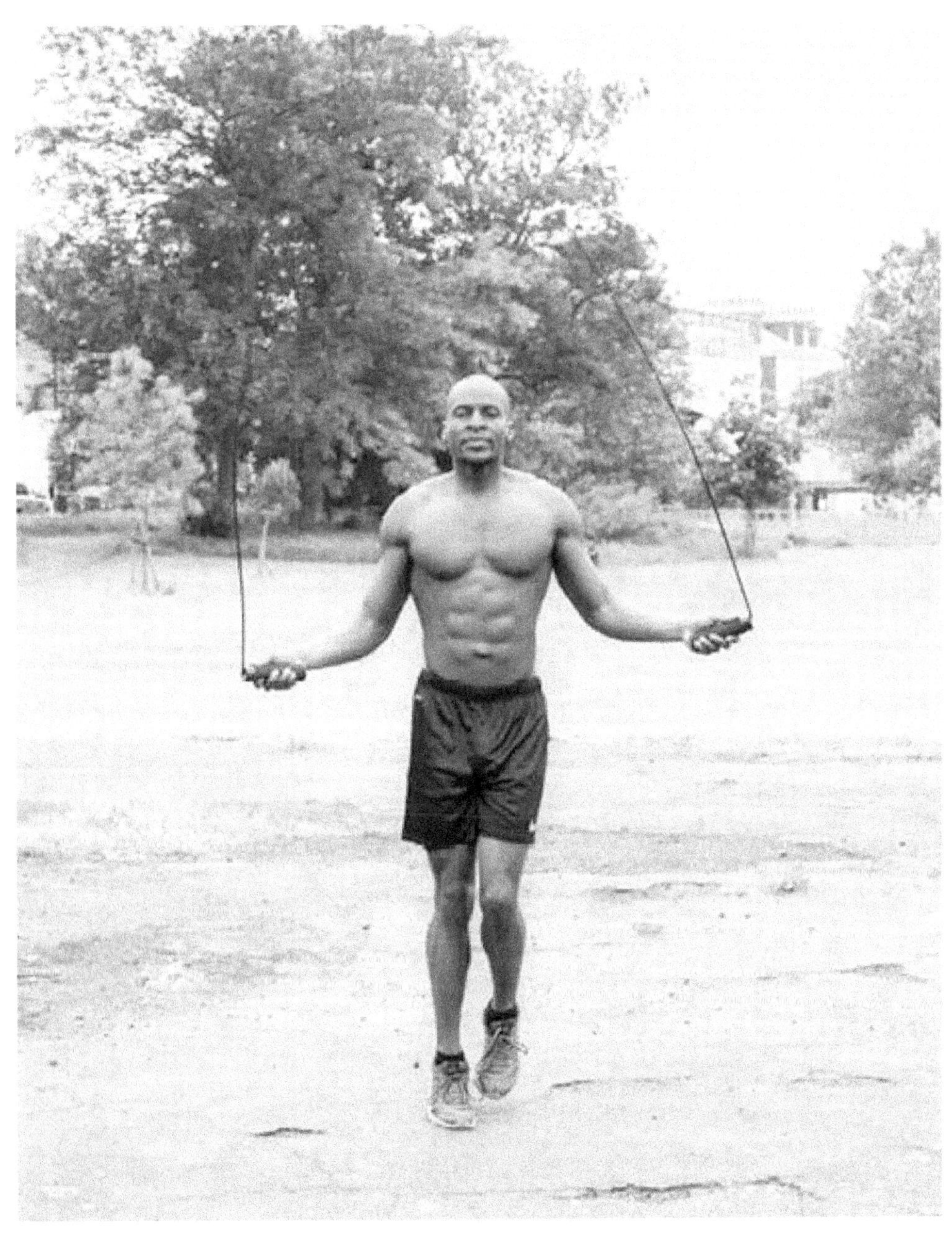

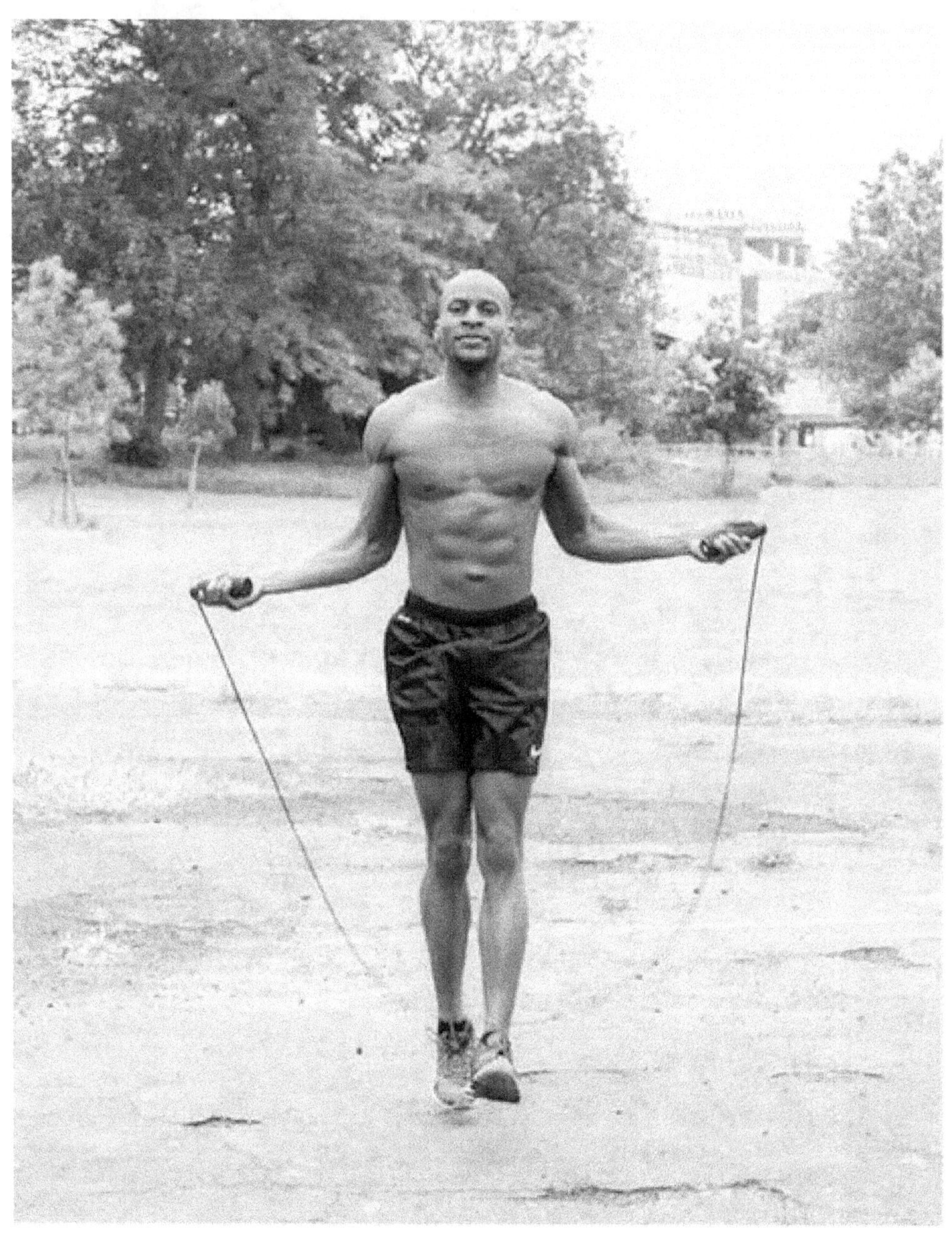

OTHER

You can probably see a trend building with cardio and conditioning – intense bursts of activity, followed by a short rest before going in all over again.

Cycling, rowing, boxing, circuits, swimming etc. are other great ways to get the blood pumping so don't be afraid to throw your own interests and hobbies into the mix.

It is generally recommended to perform 30-60 minutes of cardio per day. In addition to the benefits you already know of, you may also experience a myriad of other pros. These include reduced stress and anxiety, clarity of thought, improved sleep and even a potent antidote to depression. It really pays, then, to find a way to get your fix.

So long as your heart is pounding and your brow is dripping, you are doing cardio. It doesn't have to be by the book, but it does have to be done, and it does have to be tough. That is non-negotiable for those seeking SUPERHUMAN status.

Our mantra is simple: train hard. Two words that need to be etched into your mind whenever you enter the field of battle. Do not turn up to participate, turn up to WIN!

If you are training solo, every day should be an endeavor to reach a personal best or achieve something new. If you have a training buddy, push each other to higher levels by competing on every exercise. You will be shocked at just how far this takes you.

So, with that final gut-busting burst of activity we conclude this complete rundown of calisthenics exercises. You now possess the very same knowledge as the elite.

You have witnessed the unparalleled power of bodyweight exercise, and you have step-by-step instructions to achieve the body of your dreams.

Depending on your current level of ability, you may be ready to dive in at the deep end, or you might have to flip right back to the beginning and start at square one.

Our one key piece of advice is to understand and accept your level, and progress at your own pace. It is far more beneficial to make steady progress with proper form than it is to rush ahead and completely fail to achieve your objectives.

Flip the page for more advice on progressing with calisthenics.